Storying Domestic Violence

Frontiers of Narrrative

SERIES EDITOR
David Herman
Ohio State University

Storying Domestic Violence

Constructions and Stereotypes of Abuse
in the Discourse of General Practitioners

Jarmila Mildorf

UNIVERSITY OF NEBRASKA PRESS • LINCOLN AND LONDON

Source acknowledgments
for
previously published material
appear on p. xiv. ¶
© 2007 by the
Board of Regents
of the
University of Nebraska

¶ Library of Congress
Cataloging-in-Publication Data
¶ Mildorf, Jarmila.
¶ Storying domestic violence :
constructions and stereotypes of abuse
in the discourse of general practitioners
/ Jarmila Mildorf.
¶ p. ; cm. —
(Frontiers of narrative)
¶ Includes
bibliographical references
and index.
¶ ISBN-13: 978-0-8032-3259-4
(cloth : alk. paper)
¶ ISBN-10: 0-8032-3259-4
(cloth : alk. paper)
¶ 1. Family violence.
2. Discourse analysis, Narrative.
3. Narrative medicine.
4. Physician and patient.
5. Physicians (General practice)
I. Title. II. Series.
[DNLM: 1. Physician-Patient Relations.
2. Domestic Violence.
3. Narration.
4. Truth Disclosure.
W 62 M641S 2007]
RA1122.M55   2007
362.82'92dc—22
¶ 2006023849
¶ Set in Quadraat
& Quadraat Sans by
Kim Essman.
Designed by R. W. Boeche.

For my parents and the best sisters in the world, Jana and Julia

Contents

Preface   ix

Acknowledgments   xiii

Transcription Conventions   xv

1. Introduction   1

2. Narrative
   Theoretical Background   10

3. Domestic Violence and the Role of General Practice
   A Narrative-Analytic Approach   28

4. Signs of Abuse
   "Classic" Disclosures and Narrative Trajectories   49

5. Setting the Scene of Abuse
   Metaphors and Spatiotemporal Mapping   68

6. Mythologizing Time, Mythologizing Violence
   Backgrounds and Explanations of Domestic Abuse   94

7. Agents of Their Own Victimization
   The Women's Role in the GPs' Narratives   123

8. Evaluating Abuse
   Storied Knowledge and Salient Facts   144

9. Conclusion   173

   Appendix   187

   Notes   213

   Bibliography   219

   Index   233

Preface

Between one quarter and half of all women in the world experience domestic violence at some point in their lives, according to World Bank figures (Bunch 1997:42). Local surveys and studies throughout the world confirm this finding. Since domestic violence causes both acute physical injuries and long-term chronic illness, abused women are likely to appeal to their family doctors or general practitioners as one of their first resources for help. However, general practitioners rarely report domestic violence in their practices. Why do doctors not notice domestic violence, and why do women not disclose it to them? What makes communication about domestic violence between doctor and patient so difficult? This study's unique contribution to the problem of prevalence and oversight is its examination of doctors' narrative practices around treatment rather than the women's stories of abuse, which have received more attention in previous research. In addition, the study proposes solutions from within the same narrative paradigm.

A few studies over the last years have focused on general practitioners' attitudes toward and perceptions of domestic violence and have also, albeit mostly cursorily, taken into account stigmatizing discourses and stereotypical imagery. By considering general practitioners' narrative discourses about domestic violence against the background of theories of narrative and knowledge and by applying narrative-analytic tools, this study opens up new vistas for the application of narrative research in this field. The book has emerged from two of my main areas of interest: the relationship between language and social problems, on the one hand, and the study of narrative, on the other. As a result, this work seeks to answer two interrelated questions: first, to what extent and in what ways are notions of "language," "discourse," and "narrative" relevant for the functioning of social life and of people's everyday social practices in general as well as for the emergence and recurrence of social problems in particular? Second, can linguistic analysis and the study of narrative forms in discourse contribute to the understanding and solution of social problems? Narrative research has gained currency in a number of disciplines over the last four decades, and it has increasingly informed interdisciplinary approaches. This study demonstrates how microlevel structural analyses of narratives can be linked to cognitive and sociocultural dimensions or macrolevels of narratives and thus how narrative analysis can be operationalized for the social sciences.

The data used for the analyses were generated in in-depth interviews with twenty general practitioners in and around the city of Aberdeen, Scotland. Since in my view domestic violence is a universal phenomenon the root problems of which are not necessarily determined by local particularities, the study constitutes a case study that should be useful for researchers and interested readers anywhere in the world. Aberdeen is in many ways comparable to other cities. Situated in northeastern Scotland and home to a population of 212,125, it is a cosmopolitan port of approximately 184 square kilometers that functions as a major retail, leisure, cultural, and educational center in the country. Traditional industries such as fishing and farming still flourish in and around the city, but its economy is mainly based on the oil industry, which has earned the city a new epithet as the Oil Capital of Europe. Despite being northerly, Aberdeen is not isolated, thanks to good road, rail, sea, and air communications with other major cities and European countries. As throughout the United Kingdom, general health care is provided on a governmental level through the National Health Service (NHS), which is administered in Aberdeen by the regional health authority, the Grampian NHS Board. The Grampian NHS Board is responsible for, among other things, the health services in the Grampian region, covering primary and community care as well as hospital services, the allocation of Scottish Executive funding, and health promotion.

Sociologists, anthropologists, folklorists, linguists, sociolinguists, discourse analysts, narratologists, psychologists, and philosophers will find this interdisciplinary study interesting for theoretical and methodological reasons. While the notion that narrative encodes and conveys cultural values and attitudes that constitute and shape experience and meaning will be old news for some researchers, it is nonetheless desirable from an ethnographic point of view to address rather more than less social problems and their speech situations with sociolinguistic description. Because of its practical implications, the study is also important for policy makers, patient advocates, and health care professionals working with domestic violence. And medical humanists and medical ethicists as well as physicians themselves will benefit from an awareness of their own communication practices around an issue of great moral depth. The analyses of the GPS' narratives inevitably involve linguistic detail and terminology, but every effort has been made to keep the technical and methodological apparatus at a minimum to facilitate access and enhance readability.

Acknowledgments

I owe a great debt of gratitude to the following people: first and foremost to David Herman, without whose encouragement and trust this study would perhaps not have been turned into a book. I would also like to thank Ladette Randolph and her team at the University of Nebraska Press for their professional and rigorous work.

Furthermore, I owe great thanks to Barbara Fennell, who accompanied my research from the beginning, and to Linda McKie and Karen O'Reilly for their help and advice on research in the sociology of health and illness and domestic violence.

I would also like to thank Anna de Fina, Alan Palmer, and the anonymous reviewers of my manuscript for reading my work and for making invaluable comments and suggestions. Needless to say, all remaining shortcomings are entirely my fault. Thanks are also due to John Fowler for proofreading the book and to my copyeditor, Mary M. Hill.

The research presented in this book could not have been conducted without the financial assistance of the Faculty of Arts and Divinity and, during the initial phase of my project, the Department of General Practice & Primary Care at the University of Aberdeen.

I must also thank the twenty doctors who kindly agreed to be interviewed and thus made this project possible. I hope they will not view my work as unjust criticism but as an attempt to show ways for improving the status of domestic violence in the health care setting.

Furthermore, I wish to thank the Aberdeen Domestic Abuse Forum for letting me participate while I conducted my research. I learned a lot about the various agencies in Aberdeen that do a tremendous job in working with battered women, their children, and their violent partners.

Last but not least, I wish to express my thanks to my family and all my close friends for believing in me.

Earlier versions of parts of this book appeared in the form of journal articles, and I am grateful for permission to draw on the following:

Jarmila Mildorf, "Opening up a Can of Worms': Physicians' Narrative Construction of Knowledge about Domestic Violence," *Narrative Inquiry* 12.2 (2002). Copyright 2002 by John Benjamins. All rights reserved.

Jarmila Mildorf, "Narratives of Domestic Violence Cases: GPs Defining Their Professional Role," in Peter L. Twohig and Vera Kalitzkus, eds., *Making Sense of Health, Illness and Disease* (2004). Copyright 2004 by Rodopi. All rights reserved.

Linda McKie, Barbara Fennell, and Jarmila Mildorf, "Time to Disclose, Timing Disclosure: GPs' Discourses on Disclosing Domestic Abuse in Primary Care," *Sociology of Health and Illness* 24.3 (2002). Copyright 2002 by Blackwell. All rights reserved.

Transcription Conventions

*The transcription conventions used for this study are adopted, with slight mod-
ification, from Norrick (2000). The aim is to keep transcription symbols to a
minimum in order to enhance readability.*

Right.	Period indicates falling intonation in the preceding element.
What am I going to do here?	Question mark indicates question with or without rising intonation.
I had, er, a girl who	Comma indicates a continuing intonation, drawing out the preceding element.
^so nice	Arrowhead pointing upward indicates stress on the following element.
in ——[insight]	A 2-em dash indicates that a speaker stopped speaking midword or midsentence.
Say, "Well, you should leave him"	Double quotation marks show speech set off by a shift in the speaker's voice.
{ }	Curly braces on successive lines mark the beginning and end of overlapping talk.
[laughs] drug [user]	Square brackets enclose editorial comments or elements whose transcription is not entirely certain.
[?]	A question mark within square brackets indicates that the recording is unclear.
=	Equals signs on successive lines indicate latching between turns.
. . .	Ellipsis points indicate faltering speech.
—	An em dash indicates a sudden break in speech.
Saturday night ritual	Boldface type is used throughout extracts taken from the narratives to highlight items discussed in the text. In the appendix the narratives are marked by boldface type.

Storying Domestic Violence

1. Introduction

I'm sure there's lots of individual factors that makes people stay with
people that abuse them. And it's very difficult to tease them out.
Um, if I, I mean I would never ever ever advise anybody to stay in
that relationship. I just think that's just daft. I remember the first
time I saw it, quite cl——. **I can still vividly remember the first time
I came across a girl who'd been beaten by a guy and I was working
in casualty. She was just a young girl and he'd, I [was] just newly
qualified, and this guy had hit her. And I said, [?] he had the house
keys. Now then I said: "Could I have the house keys, please?" She
wanted her flat keys. [And I said she wanted to be?] she just wanted
to be here at the moment. And he got really, really, quite aggressive
with me. And, fortunately there was police around and they got the
keys and everything off him and, er, sat him down and told him to
behave himself. I had a long chat with her, and she left with him.
You know, she went back to him. I said: "Look, he's done that and
you've forgiven him for once, he'll do it again to ya." And you just,
I just wonder what happened, you know. But, you know, I thought,
you know, if you let him do it this once he'll always think he can
get away with it again. And, she obviously, I don't know, I don't
know why she went back.**

Young female GP from an Aberdeen city center practice

This story related by a young female GP working in a city center practice in Aberdeen, Scotland, voices some of the frustration and helplessness of medical doctors when faced with patients who suffer domestic abuse from their partners.[1]
In this emotional story the GP aligns herself with the patient and shows their
affinity in youth and inexperience. Both women in this story suffer from an
abusive man: the young woman who was beaten by her partner and the young

doctor who is verbally abused by the same man while trying to examine and treat the woman. The story becomes vivid and more "dramatic" through the use of direct speech, and it illustrates the young doctor's pang of frustration when the woman finally returns to her partner. The GP cannot understand why the woman went back, thereby echoing the frequently asked question, Why do battered women stay with the men who abuse them? Is that not "just daft," as the GP has it? This "unreasonable" behavior and the doctor's helplessness seem to be the lasting impressions that have become part of the GP's "storied knowledge" of domestic violence and that are reinforced in the storytelling situation of the interview. We learn nothing about possible reasons for the woman's decision and about how doctors can deal with this empathetically rather than dismissively. If narratives like this reproduce what doctors "know" about domestic violence, then what inferences can be made about doctors' knowledge concerning the problem? Furthermore, what do such stories tell us about domestic violence and medical practice? Like many of the other narratives in my corpus, this narrative also shows the problem of the unfinished story for the doctor: "I just wonder what happened." The beginnings of stories seem to be endlessly repeated, but one rarely gets the end of the story: abuse prevented, patient "cured." Do doctors simply not narrate, or do they also not see and intervene?

I began this book with one of the stories from the corpus for my study because it is the story of a novice's encounter with domestic violence, just as the reader at this stage is a novice to the materials I present. This is one of thirty-six narratives that emerged during interviews I conducted with general practitioners in the city of Aberdeen about their experiences with domestic violence cases. In many ways the story is typical of most of the narratives in the sample and gives a flavor of what this book is all about: it presents general practitioners' responses to domestic violence from a primarily narrative-analytic point of view; that is, it seeks to combine the investigation into a social issue with a detailed linguistic analysis of interview narratives. More precisely, this study

1. analyzes the discursive and narrative strategies general practitioners apply in interviews when they talk about their experiences with victims of domestic violence in their practice work;
2. states what these strategies reveal about GPs' perceptions of and attitudes toward domestic violence as well as about the way they

      linguistically (re)construct knowledge and realities of domestic
      violence in their narratives;

3. demonstrates what this indicates with regard to the construction of medical knowledge in general practice;

4. identifies the problems the GPs' discursive practices might reveal and, at the same time, engender for their daily work;

5. offers solutions from within the narrative framework as part of a larger endeavor to encourage cross-disciplinary collaboration.

Let me clarify these points by providing an outline of my book and by anticipating some of the central questions and answers.

Powerful discourses on a great number of topics pervade society and influence directly or indirectly, consciously or unconsciously, people's views and perceptions and thus also their sense of the world that surrounds them. As theorists such as Bourdieu (1991) maintain, language is at the heart of modern civilization, and meaning is always negotiated in people's interactions, which function largely on the basis of communication. One assumption is that discourse not only depicts reality but in fact also reproduces it by setting up parameters and conceptual frameworks according to which people judge and perceive other people and their actions as well as their own experiences (Fairclough 1992; van Dijk 1997). In this sense discourse is constitutive and constructive, and it becomes a potent commodity by which knowledge is produced and maintained and social power is seized (Foucault 1981). Likewise, narrative cannot only be regarded as a discourse mode; it is also a cognitive device that helps us order our life experiences and make sense of the world (Herman 2002). On a wider societal level stories contain the common knowledge a group of people share, and narratives thus become the storage space as well as the vehicle for transmitting cultural knowledge and wisdom (Celi and Boiero 2002). It is not least for this reason that narrative analysis has an important place in a number of current social sciences and other research areas, including artificial intelligence, cognitive and social psychology, linguistics, medical philosophy, and sociology.

As I demonstrate in chapter 2, narrative analysis in sociolinguistics has in the past contributed to the investigation of social problems and has tried to put forward possible solutions, for example, in the area of emergency calls (Imbens-Bailey and McCabe 2000) and the study of people's perceptions of the German reunification (Dittmar and Bredel 1999). However, what moves the analysis presented here beyond traditional discourse-analytic approaches such as Critical Discourse Analysis (CDA), for example, is the cognitive dimension in the investigation of narrative data. Drawing upon Herman's (1999b) concept of "socio-narratology," with its emphasis on linguistic, contextual, and cognitive factors in narrative production, I analyze the GPs' narratives not only with regard to their linguistic form and the situational context in which they were produced but also with a view to identifying the cognitive processes that might underlie and inform these narratives. The assumption that a link can be established between GPs' knowledge of domestic violence and the way they relate case stories mainly draws upon the theoretical background of Bruner's (1986), Sarbin's (1986), and Schank's (1990) work on narrative thinking and narrative knowledge, which I discuss in chapter 2. The questions raised for my study are, How can one establish a link between macrolevel and microlevel structures or, in this specific context, between GPs' narrative discourses and the cognitive processes by which they conceptualize and understand domestic violence? What do the narratives reveal about doctors' knowledge of the problem? From a sociolinguistic standpoint the aim of this study is to emphasize the *social* side of the discipline by applying discourse-analytic techniques to a social problem with real-life implications. By emphasizing *narrative* in this study I test the applicability of narrative tools to a social problem and thus not only provide further insights in the area of narrative research but point toward solutions to the problem from within the narrative framework.

As I argue throughout the book, narrative stands out as a special discursive device because it attends to particularities and detail in people's experiences. It offers a special way of ordering events and experiences in a person's memory and also of recounting them to other people. Narrative forms the basis for the way people make sense of and give meaning to their lives by imposing ordered narrative structures on what would otherwise be perceived as chaotic life experiences. By indexing and storing narratives in their memories, people also compile what Polkinghorne (1995) calls "storied knowledge" about other people, events, experiences, and so on. This storied knowledge can be retrieved at any time when the situation requires such specific information. Narrative is also a successful and popular discursive device, I argue, because it is engaging and often entertaining, which makes it ideal for negotiating and exchanging ideas, life experiences, values, attitudes, and feelings. If we consider the way the news media, for example, employ narrative structures, it becomes obvious that one big advantage narrative has over other discursive devices is the fact that it can be captivating and that it is more suitable for the expression of affective meaning, for example. Narrative also offers us an indirect and therefore less threatening way of conveying our opinions and values. In a sense, narrators can "hide behind" the story they tell, and thus narratives are less confrontational than other forms of discourse. If we accept the premise that narrative constitutes as well as (re-)creates knowledge and the reality people perceive, then the GPS' narratives about their experiences with patients who suffer domestic violence also reveal their perceptions of the issue and, at the same time, reinforce a certain "reality" of domestic violence cases in their minds. In chapter 2 I also discuss to what extent doctors draw upon narrative knowledge constituted by stories about patients and cases.

It is not surprising then that almost all the GPS I interviewed related narratives at least once during the interview. Some GPS repeatedly resumed the same narrative, while others told me more than one. Some of the narratives can be regarded as fully fledged narratives in the Labovian sense (i.e., they follow largely the diamond diagram of narratives, which I outline in chapter 3), while others appear abbreviated or are not fully expanded upon. This may be attributed to the restrictions imposed by the interview format. Equally important in this context are questions of politeness (Brown and Levinson 1987) as well as the Gricean maxims of relevance and brevity, which I explain in more detail in chapter 3. Ultimately, any dialogue must be regarded as "talk-in-interaction," during which participants collaborate to have a successful conversation. Likewise, oral narratives are always coconstructions between storyteller and listener or narrator and narratee, respectively, another guiding assumption in my study.

Since narratives are never related in a vacuum but are always situated in a special linguistic and interactional context and are told to other people for a specific purpose (Schiffrin 1993; Schegloff 1997; Imbens-Bailey and McCabe 2000; Norrick 2000), the analysis of narratives requires a theoretical framework that incorporates the notion of complex layers of interaction. In the frame model that I propose in chapter 3 the interactional character of a joint narrative production within the interview frame is captured by embedded frames of expectations and of rules for interaction. The two frames considered in the actual analyses of the GPS' narratives are the narrative frame and the interview frame. The narrative frame imposes rules and expectations concerning the structural and thematic elaboration of narratives and the roles of narrator and narratee in narrative production. The interview frame is equally important in this context, as it also sets up behavioral rules for the interaction between interviewer and interviewee. In my analyses I take account of these influential factors by paying close attention to features typical of talk-in-interaction. Thus I discuss hesitation markers, defensive answers, self-criticism, politeness features, phatic features, and high-involvement style. As the analyses reveal, the GPS were aware of the interview situation and therefore accommodated their speech in order to maintain face as well as to allow myself as the interviewer to maintain face (Goffman 1967; Giles and Smith 1979). Some GPS chose their words with care, as could be seen in a number of self-monitoring devices. In sum, the influence of the mechanisms of interpersonal perception (Laing, Phillipson, and Lee 1966) and various expectations based on differences in gender, age, and status could sometimes be felt and observed in the GPS' discourses. After all, I was not a colleague whose moral trajectory could be assumed and a woman whose feminist agenda might be hidden. All this is explained more fully, for example, in chapters 7 and 9. In one narrative that I discuss in chapter 9 silence also in a way enacts on a discursive level a strategy often adopted in society: to collude with the victims' silence rather than to challenge abuse. The question of taboos and of "unspeakable" stories is thus another crucial point in my book.

As I discuss in chapter 4, one of the problems emerging from the GPS' narratives is that of divergent narrative trajectories in doctors' and patients' stories. A lot of the narratives in my sample are "incomplete" in that they either leave out the women's stories (e.g., what their personal backgrounds were, how they experienced the violence, etc.) or lack closure in the sense that either violence is prevented or treatment proves successful. I discuss this finding somewhat flippantly by contending that what is missing in the GPS' narratives is "hero stories." Perhaps we cannot expect medical doctors to find "cures" for domestic violence. We can, however, expect them to be receptive enough to keep the gates to salient help resources open. For this purpose it is essential that medical narratives, with their mostly linear trajectory of presentation–diagnosis–treatment–cure, converge more strongly with battered women's life narratives, which may not follow the same pattern. In chapter 3 I present statistical studies that reveal that GPs frequently miss cases partly because they lack the necessary sensitivity to hidden signs of abuse. In addition, feminist researchers have focused on ideological issues surrounding the perpetuation of male-defined cultural myths and stigmatizing discourses. While all these studies offer great insights, there has hitherto been no research that illuminated the microlevel linguistic mechanisms by which doctors (re-)create discourses and concepts on domestic violence. Through its primarily linguistic focus and detailed narrative analyses this study therefore closes a gap in this particular research area. I argue that one way of working toward improvement in the disclosure and subsequent treatment of domestic violence cases is by erasing the mismatch between doctors' and patients' expectations, views, and attitudes, which manifest themselves in their divergent narratives and narrative practices. This process needs to commence in people's minds.

I already indicated that my study is an interdisciplinary endeavor and as such draws upon insights and research from a number of disciplines as varied as sociolinguistics and discourse studies, sociology, social and cognitive psychology, narratology, and philosophy. Since the narrative paradigm is the overarching framework that holds together my various approaches and analyses, I begin by providing a theoretical discussion of the significance of narrative in people's lives and its treatment in various disciplines in chapter 2. In the third chapter I provide further background information to my study by surveying the literature on domestic violence in the health care setting. This allows me to highlight some of the complexities in doctor-patient interaction surrounding domestic violence that have already been identified in the literature and also to demonstrate in what ways the narrative-analytic approach I adopt here can enhance our understanding of these complexities. In chapter 4 I introduce data from my sample that function as "normalizing data" to the actual narratives I analyze in subsequent chapters. These largely nonnarrative data from the interviews provide kinds of information that are missing from much of the narrative material, for example, with regard to signs of abuse and "typical" scenarios. I discuss this discrepancy by looking at the concept of narrative trajectories, which has played a major role in life narrative research. After this fairly general approach to my data I then undertake close linguistic analyses of the GPs' narratives by investigating four major areas: spatiotemporal mapping and metaphors in chapter 5; the mythologizing of time in general practice and of backgrounds and explanations of abuse in chapter 6; agency and the role of social as well as professional actors from the perspective of both the woman and the doctor in chapter 7; and, finally, the GPs' evaluation of both the severity and significance of domestic violence cases in chapter 8. In narratological terms I move from a discussion of circumstantial narrative matters, or the "setting," to a presentation of the narratives' "characters" and then to the narrator's "point of view." Detailed analyses of linguistic features such as spatiotemporal language, metaphors, modalities, thematic roles, and active/passive constructions as well as evaluative devices are the tools for unraveling the mechanisms that set up GPs' conceptual explanatory frameworks about domestic violence. The conclusion in chapter 9 pulls together these various strings and demonstrates in a summary to what extent the diverse approaches of the previous chapters yield overlapping results. I show how the GPs reveal their perceptions of and attitudes toward domestic violence in their narratives and to what extent these might be problematic. More important, however, as this study uniquely illuminates these issues as a wider problem of narrative practices, I will then point in the direction of possible solutions that narrative analysis has to offer for medical training. Since the value of narrative discourse for both practitioner and care recipient is increasingly acknowledged in the medical setting, a good case can be made for the type of narrative-analytic "take" I propose here.

Before I move on to the discussion of the theoretical background to this study I need to clarify some of the terms that will be used throughout and that also imply my own position. No research takes place in a vacuum, and the interpretation of data is always influenced by the particular cultural, sociohistorical, and political lens through which the researcher views the data. I refer to battered women as "victims" in acknowledgment of the fact that domestic violence is overwhelmingly perpetrated by men on women and because I believe that domestic violence, whatever its individual reasons and circumstances, is ultimately also a result of a wider imbalance of power and inequality between men and women and of still latent misogynist attitudes in society. I am aware that the term has also been contested by feminist researchers, as it potentially frames abused women as helpless and passive (Lamb 1999). This is not the way I want to use it here. "Cultural myths" about domestic violence refer to a number of preconceived ideas about the problem that I discuss in greater detail in chapter 3. The underlying assumption is that "knowledge" of domestic violence is also constructed in and through the discourses of individuals, advocates, institutions, the media, and so on. Hence I use the term *discourse* in Foucault's (1981, 1982) sense as an intersection where knowledge is produced and maintained and thus becomes a site for constant power struggles. This "macrostructural" level of ideas and conceptions of domestic violence is interrelated with the "microstructural" level of actual discussions and discursive practices.

Finally, I do not consider "stereotypes" a priori as distortions of reality, that is, as negative, as is often the case in common parlance and in some of the social psychology literature on the issue. On the contrary, I follow McGarty, Yzerbyt, and Spears (2002) in assuming that stereotypes are sets of "relations between knowledge, labels and perceived equivalences" (McGarty 2002:18) whose primary function is to provide explanatory systems and to form meaningful beliefs about social groups. Stereotype formation is a context-dependent dynamic process that allows groups to develop tools *"both to represent their members' shared social reality and to achieve particular objectives within it"* (Haslam et al. 2002:161, emphasis in original). As my discussion of the GPS' narratives demonstrates, a problem arises when stereotypes of victims and perpetrators of domestic abuse are oversimplified and lead to one-sided pictures of the problem. Let me now provide an overview of narrative research traditions and the theoretical framework to my study.

2. Narrative

Theoretical Background

There is no knowing without theory, that is, a set of assumptions and categories that can be tested and then reformulated or modified through further theorizing. As the literary critic Terry Eagleton puts it: "All of our descriptive statements move within an often invisible network of value-categories, and indeed without such categories we would have nothing to say to each other at all" (1996:12). In order to clarify how I arrived at my results I need to say first what questions and assumptions concerning narrative guided my research. I will accomplish this in this chapter, in which I first consider the relationship between narrative and social problems, then narrative as an intrinsic human feature and activity, and finally narrative as a special discursive element in the medical setting.

Narrative and Social Problems

Stories have formed part of any culture known to us. Anthropologists point out that for hundreds of years stories have ensured the survival and passing down of knowledge and beliefs (Celi and Boiero 2002; Kirmayer 2000). As Celi and Boiero contend in their study on Native American narratives, stories are a vehicle for conveying knowledge:

> Poetic storytelling presents to our imagination something that resembles the human actions with which we are directly acquainted through experience. Stories are composed of the knowledge people share and this shared knowledge serves as a vital base that has the potential to help them discover meaning in other contexts. . . . Stories do more than delight us and give us pleasure; they certainly instruct in a manner that is comparable to the instruction we receive from works of science, philosophy, theology, history and biography. (2002:61)

In a similar vein Herman defines narrative not only as a discourse genre but also as a "cognitive style," and he contends that "stories both have a logic and are a logic in their own right" (2002:22); that is, narratives not only are structured in specific ways in order to be understood but also constitute a "logic by virtue of which people (including writers) know when, how, and why to use stories to enable themselves and others to find their way in the world" (2002:24). Put differently, stories serve concrete functions (e.g., to make or illustrate a point, to convey a moral, etc.), and we generally know when to use such stories.

The notion that language plays an essential role in social life and therefore in the social sciences has had a long tradition in linguistics. An early example are Edward Sapir's influential ideas about language and environment, which were further elaborated by Sapir's student, Benjamin Lee Whorf, and which have become known in linguistics as the Sapir-Whorf hypothesis. The main argument is that the language one uses and that is the expression of one's culture essentially shapes one's view of the world.[1] Although Sapir recognized the importance of the study of language for a better understanding of social reality as early as the late 1920s, it was not until the 1960s that the relationship among language, social structures, and social problems started to be systematically investigated and thus gave rise to a "new" branch of linguistics, namely, *socio*linguistics. Ever since, the application of linguistic expertise has not only provided deeper insights into social problems but often assisted in solving these problems.[2] In the 1980s linguists' interest in the relationship between language and social problems reached a first peak. For example, in 1988 the journal *Social Problems* dedicated a special issue to the relationship among language, interaction, and social problems. The editor and one of the authors in this special issue, Maynard (1988), emphasizes that a language-oriented social science that pays special attention to the organization of the interaction order can matter significantly to scholars' understanding of social problems and the sociology of deviance. In other words, the analysis of people's linguistic interactions can contribute to the understanding of wider social issues, since linguistic interactions are at the heart of these issues.[3] The argument is that social structures manifest themselves in the sequential organization of linguistic interaction to the extent that interactants display their awareness of and sensitivity to the situational context in which the interaction takes place and, accordingly, accommodate their speech (Wilson 1991:37). As a consequence, language not only offers tools for

forming different types of interaction (e.g., storytelling) but is equally shaped
by already existing preconceptions and expectations to which speakers orien-
tate themselves. It is in this sense that narrative interaction reinforces and, at
the same time, reconstructs social structures.

A research area where the sequential analysis of talk has been applied and
has foregrounded problems is the analysis of emergency calls (Whalen, Zimmerman, and Whalen 1988). Imbens-Bailey and McCabe (2000) approach the
problem by applying sociolinguistic narrative analysis. They argue that calls to
the emergency department "share key components with the typical narrative
genre" (Imbens-Bailey and McCabe 2000:289), for example, orientation information and complicating actions that relate the nature of the emergency.[4] However, the discrepancy between narrative form and the requirements imposed
on emergency calls may lead to communication problems and subsequent lack
of salient help provision: "The descriptions of events in an emergency call are
constrained by their dual functions of maximizing the speedy transfer of vital information while minimizing the inclusion of superfluous detail. It is this
trade off between concerns such as efficiency and the urge to narrate human
experience that may contribute to an inherent communicative tension in placing a 911 call" (Imbens-Bailey and McCabe 2000:289). Clearly, Imbens-Bailey
and McCabe consider narrative a fundamental device in human communication that is used daily by speakers to convey their meaning to others. Narrative
is more than a discursive device, however. In fact, it can be argued that narrative pervades human thinking and thus resembles other acts of comprehension,
as Robinson and Hawpe contend: "Stories are a means for interpreting or rein-
terpreting events by constructing a causal pattern which integrates that which
is known about an event as well as that which is conjectural but relevant to an
interpretation" (1986:112).

Research conducted in Germany offers a poignant example of the way narrative interaction and the construction of social structures are related. Dittmar
and Bredel (1999) analyzed in their study of East and West Berliners' narratives
about the fall of the Berlin wall on November 9, 1989, how the historical events
of that night had been perceived and also related differently by people from the
eastern and western parts of the city. Moreover, Dittmar and Bredel showed to
what extent the narratives (re)constructed images and stereotypes of "Ossis"
and "Wessis" (i.e., East Germans and West Germans), which even ten years af-

ter reunification created a distance between easterners and westerners and thus impeded a successful integration of the two former Germanys. This example demonstrates in what ways linguistic narrative research not only helps unravel social problems but also offers possible solutions. By compiling their data in a narrative corpus that is also available on the internet, Dittmar and Bredel set up a "collective memory" that could be used for discussions in the classroom, for example, and ideally raise awareness about people's perceptions and the discursive strategies by which they convey their perceptions.

Labov and Waletzky's (1967) groundbreaking article "Narrative Analysis: Oral Versions of Personal Experience" is probably the most significant example of the growing interest in narrative structure in the 1960s. This article has been very influential and initiated a whole subdiscipline within the area of sociolinguistics, the extent of which is captured in the special issue of the *Journal of Narrative and Life History* published in 1997 (Bamberg 1997), in which eminent scholars from various disciplines reflect on thirty years of narrative analysis. Although this collection gives the impression that the study of narratives has finally become an interdisciplinary endeavor, there was relatively little cross-fertilization between disciplines until almost two decades after Labov and Waletzky's article. In the eighties the need for a "contextualist narratology" (Tolliver 1997) was felt and expressed by narratologists and linguists alike (Lanser 1981; Farrell 1985), and attempts were made to systematically integrate linguistic and literary approaches to narrative (Fludernik 1996; Kanyó 1986; Toolan 2001).

The second theoretical pillar of my study, Herman's (1999b) concept of "socionarratology," has emerged from traditional narratology, which was influenced by French structuralism and set in motion as a more systematic discipline after the appearance of the English translation of Vladimir Propp's (1968) morphological study of fairy tales.[5] Herman's innovative, integrated approach offers a conceptual model that "situates stories in a constellation of linguistic, cognitive, and contextual factors" (1999b:219). In his analysis of oral ghost stories Herman includes notions and methods from classical narratology, conversation analysis, and interactional sociolinguistics to illuminate the context in which the stories were told. The underlying assumption is that narrativeness, or "narrativehood," as Herman puts it, requires more than specific structural properties: "What makes a story a story cannot be ascribed to narrative form alone, but rather arises from the interplay between the semantic content of the narrative; the formal features of the discourse through which such narrated content manifests itself; and the kinds of inferences promoted via this interplay of form and content in particular discourse contexts" (1999b:229). In a vacuum narratives, like language in general, do not really "mean" anything. Narratives must be told to someone for a purpose. By taking into account the functional and contextual dimensions Herman adds more depth to his concept, and it thus proves a good working model for the kinds of narratives I analyze in this study.

Homo narrans; or, Why Do We Tell Stories?

The subtitle of a special feature in the *Journal of Communications* 35.4, "*Homo Narrans*: Story-Telling in Mass Culture and Everyday Life," suggests that storytelling is an intrinsically human characteristic, much as language as such seems to be a biological faculty most highly developed in the human species (Chomsky 1988; Pinker 1994, 1997). Rhetorician Walter Fisher borrows the term *Homo narrans* from Plato and uses it in his description of the "narrative paradigm," which "can be considered a dialectical synthesis of two traditional strands in the history of rhetoric: the argumentative, persuasive theme and the literary, aesthetic theme" (1984:2). In Fisher's view the narrative paradigm competes nowadays with the scientific paradigm and thus with a discourse of technical reasoning. The great contest for the *logos*, that is, the competition between the narrative and the scientific paradigm as to which one will dominate public discourse, has "contributed to the contemporary condition by repressing the realization of a holistic sense of self, by subverting the formulation of a humane concept of rationality and a sane praxis, by rendering personal and public decision making and action subservient to 'experts' in knowledge, truth, and reality, and by elevating one class of persons and their discourse over others" (Fisher 1985:87). Fisher proposes the narrative paradigm as a model that reunites the different components of discourse in the conceptualization of human beings as storytellers. The narrative paradigm also becomes a theoretical framework for the analysis of how people create social realities. Fisher contrasts the concept of storytelling as an intrinsic human characteristic with dramatism as it is proposed in Goffman's (1974) frame theory, for example:

> Dramatism *implies* a prescribed role for people; they are actors performing roles constrained or determined by scripts provided by ex-

isting institutions. The narrative paradigm sees people as storytell-ers—authors and co-authors who creatively read and evaluate the texts of life and literature. It envisions existing institutions as pro-viding "plots" that are always in the process of re-creation rather than as scripts; it stresses that people are full participants in the making of messages, whether they are agents (authors) or audience members (co-authors). (1985:86)

I argue that dramatism and the narrative paradigm need not necessarily ex-clude each other. On the contrary, these two concepts seem to have the poten-tial to act as complementary theorems in an interactional narrative theory that views narrative production as a joint project undertaken by speakers in a set-ting that is influenced equally by social and institutional rules. This approach can prove particularly useful in studies such as the one presented here, in which informants are not only individuals but also representatives of a specific pro-fessional and therefore institutional group, in this case medical doctors. The question of narrative discourse in this wider social context thus also assumes sociopolitical dimensions, as it has implications for current medical practice and for medical training.

As I mentioned above, the notion of *Homo narrans* presupposes storytelling as an innate human characteristic. Research on narratives by aphasics indeed seems to suggest that sentence-level surface devices, which are located along with other language features in certain parts of the brain, have an important function in the creation of hierarchical and evaluative structures in narratives (Ulatowska and Streit Olness 1997). However, whether this mainly biological explanation gives a complete picture or whether other factors such as culture and the socialization process also have parts to play in narrative production re-mains debatable and calls for more extensive research in this field. At any rate, there can be no doubt that telling stories forms an essential part of human in-teraction. Whether children tell their parents stories about what they have ex-perienced, or parents couch lessons about what is right or wrong in the form of fairy tales and other narratives, or we tell our friends, roommates, or part-ners in the evening about what has happened to us during the day, or we throw in personal stories while we discuss topics with other people, narratives play a significant role in our everyday lives and form an elementary basis of our daily conversations with others.

Sarbin identifies narrative as a root metaphor for psychology and considers the narratory principle, that is, the fact that "human beings think, perceive, imagine, and make moral choices according to narrative structures" (1986:8), an organizing principle in human thought essential for survival in modern society: "The rituals of daily life are organized to tell stories. The pageantry of rites of passage and rites of intensification are storied actions. Our plannings, our rememberings, even our loving and hating, are guided by narrative plots. The claim that the narratory principle facilitates survival must be taken seriously. Survival in a world of meanings is problematic without the talent to make up and to interpret stories about interweaving lives" (1986:11). Put differently, personal narratives, with their fairly conventional spatiotemporal structures, help us order our otherwise chaotic experiences of life as constant flux and passing. The argument that narratives facilitate orientation in a bureaucratic world sounds perfectly plausible if we consider language a symbolic system within which values are negotiated. Or, to adopt Bourdieu's metaphoric image of the marketplace, "linguistic exchange . . . is also an economic exchange which is established within a particular symbolic relation of power between a producer, endowed with a certain linguistic capital, and a consumer (or a market), and which is capable of procuring a certain material or symbolic profit" (1991:66). The "profit" that discourse can yield manifests itself, for example, in power and authority. Narrative as one of many discursive devices consequently also participates in the symbolic marketplace, and we can infer that people who successfully employ the narrative mode to convey their meanings and to achieve their goals have a better standing in our linguistically encoded society.

The political and institutional power of discourse has been explored, for example, by researchers in *Critical Discourse Analysis* (Titscher et al. 2000). As Fairclough points out, "power in discourse is to do with powerful participants *controlling and constraining the contributions of non-powerful participants*" (1989:46, emphasis in original). Discourse influences people's perceptions of other people, and it thus becomes a potent tool in establishing power relations: "Having the power to determine things like which word meanings or which linguistic and communicative norms are legitimate or 'correct' or 'appropriate' is an important aspect of social and ideological power, and therefore a focus of ideological struggle" (Fairclough 1989:88–89).[6] Political, legal, educational, and other institutions in any given society are thus in a powerful position, as they determine to a large extent which discourses are acceptable and made available to people. As far as the medical setting is concerned, it is overwhelmingly the case that doctors' discourse is more powerful than patients' discourse, particularly in a society in which professional expertise is highly valued. If we accept the premise that GPs' discourse ultimately has an impact on the way they work, then a close analysis of their discourse is imperative for understanding dynamic processes in general practice.

A lot of medical doctors' work can also be viewed in terms of a "ritual," in Sarbin's sense, by means of which patients and doctors try to establish the cause of the problem presented in the consultation. The way GPs often explain procedures while they perform an examination can also take a narrative form, especially if the GP has to translate technical terms into the language of the layperson. For patients, storytelling can even become a means of reclaiming power in doctor-patient communication, as Ainsworth-Vaughn argues, and stories play a crucial role in diagnosis: "Patients use the 'Why I'm here' narrative to set the scene for diagnoses; they suggest candidate diagnoses (diagnostic storyworlds), they offer evidence for and against possible diagnostic storyworlds, and they may even challenge physicians' conclusions as to the correct diagnostic storyworld" (1998:169). Strong (1979) talks about the "ceremonial order" in consultations, that is, a medical frame in which both doctor and patient act out their expected roles and try to reach a satisfying and agreeable conclusion to their conversation. However, communication between doctor and patient and subsequent provision of salient help can be impeded if doctors' and patients' narratives do not match: "While, to some extent, differences in narrative are inevitable between the clinician (a well person) and the patient (inhabiting illness), problems arise when clinicians use their disease-category narratives to dominate patients' illness narratives to such an extent that the patients' [narratives] are obliterated, leaving them demoralised, and sometimes, misdiagnosed" (Donald 1998:23–24). It is to such mismatches in doctors' and patients' narratives that I will turn in my analyses.

Moreover, narratives seem to hold an important place in people's assertions of who they are, what they do, and why they do it, in short, their identity. Linguists, sociologists, and psychologists alike have repeatedly emphasized the role that narrative construction plays in establishing identity (Johnstone 1990; Schiffrin 1996; Antaki and Widdicombe 1998; Crossley 2000; De Fina, Schiffrin, and Bamberg 2006). Furthermore, stories are essentially performative and are often used strategically in order to establish group identity and to reinforce or challenge the status quo of a group's values and beliefs, as Langellier and Peterson (2004) demonstrate in their study on family storytelling in Franco-American families. On an individual level we can argue with Schank that "we are the stories we like to tell" (1990:137), and we gradually become the stories that we like to tell often. Stories in that sense also constitute an important factor for self-understanding: "We tell stories to describe ourselves not only so others can understand who we are but also so we can understand ourselves. Telling our stories allows us to compile our personal mythology, and the collection of stories we have compiled is to some extent who we are, what we have to say about the world, and tells the world the state of our mental health" (Schank 1990:44). People often attempt to live up to the "personal mythology" they have created about themselves (or in fact that others have created about them). Narrative psychology offers further poignant examples for the validity of Schank's contention, since in this line of therapy patients are encouraged to overcome their problems by gradually revising their self-narratives.

To come back to the argument put forth at the beginning of this chapter, we can even consider storytelling part of human knowledge, as Bruner (1986) argues in his book *Actual Minds, Possible Worlds*. If one takes into account the etymology of the word "narrate," which is cognate with the older Latin word for "knowing," *gnarus* (Rigney 1992), the connection between narration, truth, and knowledge seems to be one that ancient philosophers partly recognized but that gradually faded when narrative came to be viewed as part of the fictional and fantastic realm (Fisher 1985). Bruner distinguishes between two modes of cognitive functioning that provide distinctive ways of ordering experience and, moreover, of constructing reality.[7] On the one hand, there is what Bruner calls the "paradigmatic" or "logico-scientific" mode, which "attempts to fulfill the ideal of a formal, mathematical system of description and explanation. It employs categorization or conceptualization and the operations by which categories are established, instantiated, idealized, and related one to the other to form a system" (1986:12). On the other hand, there is the "narrative" mode, or "storied knowledge," as Polkinghorne (1995) relabeled this form of cognition. In contrast to paradigmatic cognition, narrative cognition focuses on the particular characteristics of actions and picks out a specific episode rather than trying to establish a general type. It takes into account the diversity of human behavior and "attends to the temporal context and complex interaction of the elements that make each situation remarkable" (Polkinghorne 1995:11). This narrative knowledge is maintained in stories. In exchanging narratives with other people, in our "transactions," to use another of Bruner's terms, we negotiate and constitute our knowledge and thereby create social realities. According to Bruner,

> meaning is what we can agree upon or at least accept as a working basis for seeking agreement about the concept at hand. If one is arguing about social "realities" like democracy or equity or even gross national product, the reality is not the thing, not in the head, but in the act of arguing and negotiating about the meaning of such concepts. Social realities are not bricks that we trip over or bruise ourselves on when we kick at them, but the meanings that we achieve by the sharing of human cognitions. (1986:122)

Knowledge is consequently only perceptible when people talk with others about what they know, or, as Bruner puts it, "psychological reality is revealed when a distinction made in one domain—language, modes of organizing human knowledge, whatever—can be shown to have a base in the psychological processes that people use in negotiating their transactions with the world" (1986:92). Since language is the main vehicle for conveying ideas and thoughts, discourse linguistics and, more specifically, narrative analysis prove to be valuable tools for methodically unraveling the underlying principles in forms of talk, and they are therefore useful disciplines for coming to terms with cognitive processes preceding and accompanying talk-in-interaction.

I should add the caveat here that establishing a link between conversation and cognition is not unproblematic and that it has been contested by, for example, discursive psychologists, who argue that all we can observe in conversations is what people *do* by using certain discursive strategies and what they *achieve* by doing this in the given context (te Molder and Potter 2005). I believe, however, that linguistic interaction always also involves mental functioning in the sense that interlocutors try to intuit what the other person is thinking, aiming at, suggesting, and so on and that this is also true of interactions between informants and researchers. As Sanders points out, "our 'observations' of what has occurred actually are interpretations of the discourse objects in question, as well as interpretations of relevant specifics in their environment (including the specification of what makes such specifics 'relevant')" (2005:59). In other words, what linguists and social scientists unravel by means of discourse or narrative analysis always also reflects their own interpretations of their informants' linguistic behavior and thus not only the informants' but also their own cognitive functioning in the research process. For this reason I consider it perfectly legitimate to attempt to arrive at an understanding of underlying cognitive aspects, especially if they can be tied to wider cultural considerations. In this study, for example, a close analysis of logical connectors, metaphors, modalities, and spatiotemporal mapping as well as of character presentation and evaluation in the doctors' narratives reveals both the way these GPs negotiate their views and knowledge of domestic violence with the interviewer and, ultimately, their knowledge as such. As my analyses will demonstrate, this knowledge itself is embedded in cultural assumptions concerning domestic violence that are not only reflected by but also reproduced in the GPs' narratives.

Psychologists as well as researchers in artificial intelligence have attempted to establish the relationship between storytelling and knowledge. In the late 1970s Schank and Abelson (1977) presented knowledge in terms of the "conceptual dependency theory," a theory based on notions of the interplay amongst scripts, plans, goals, and understanding. "Script" is a crucial concept in this theory. It is "a structure that describes appropriate sequences of events in a particular context. A script is made up of slots and requirements about what can fill those slots" (Schank and Abelson 1977:41). The restaurant script, for example, would contain the gist of what can be expected to happen in a restaurant: ordering food, being served by a waiter, and paying the bill at the end of the meal. Scripts offer a way of labeling and encoding very specific and detailed knowledge of certain situations in a generalized form. If people had to consciously remember every single detail that belongs to the restaurant script, for instance, their memory would be overtaxed. Instead, recurrent situations or events are indexed and stored as scripts, facilitating a later retrieval of knowledge about these situations. Understanding, then, can be viewed as "a process by which people match what they see and hear to pre-stored groupings of actions that they have already experienced. New information is understood in terms of old information" (Schank and Abelson 1977:67). Likewise, when we remember and tell stories we retrieve them from and at the same time reestablish them in our long-term memories. As Schank (1990) points out, even seemingly ad hoc narratives are stories that we have already thought about at some point and that have thus become part of the memorized stock of narratives surrounding our experience. In that sense, stories are knowledge, and in telling stories we not only recall this knowledge but actively readjust and even re-create it and thus also create reality in our minds.

As far as my interviews with the doctors are concerned, this means that, through their narratives about their experiences with domestic violence patients, GPs might also express their preconceived ideas about the issue; in short, the doctors' responses reveal what they think and know and indeed what they think they know about domestic violence. The stories doctors tell are based on cases that were in some way memorable and that have consequently been indexed and stocked in the GPs' "storied knowledge" about domestic violence. Since stories in our culture usually relate "reportable events" (Labov 1972a), that is, events that are worth telling, the doctors' narratives reflect what aspects of domestic violence cases they consider important, memorable, and worth reporting. Therefore, doctors' stories can be said to indirectly reveal their attitudes toward domestic violence and the extent of their knowledge base concerning this issue, which they have acquired through their daily work experience. However, narratives are not simply transparencies to GPs' attitudes. As the preceding discussion demonstrates, what Labov calls "narrative transformations of experience" might also be presentations of self.

Narrative and Medicine: Doctors' Stories

Language plays a crucial role in the work of medical doctors but not only with regard to doctor-patient communication. Foucault contends in his *Birth of the Clinic* (1973:95) that the perception of the body and of disease is related to the syntax of a descriptive language that comprises both signs and symptoms. In other words, disease only exists when it has been recognized and codified with the signifiers of medical discourse. As Dingwall has it: "There are no diseases in nature, merely relationships between organisms. . . . Diseases are produced by the conceptual schemes imposed on the natural world by human beings, which value some states of the body and disvalue others" (1992:165). Labeling disease, giving a name to the physical state in front of one, thus becomes an essential activity in medicine. Doctor-patient interaction in a consultation can therefore be regarded as a highly specialized linguistic situation. A major part of medical doctors' work consists of analyzing and labeling the symptoms a patient presents in a consultation. Doctors interpret the signs and then make a diagnosis.

Labeling as such often has far-reaching consequences, as Maynard (1988) maintains, because to give a name to a "trouble" or a "problem" means that one reinforces at the same time the status quo of this problem as given. Maynard exemplifies this with an extract from a dialogue between a pediatrician and a mother whose child seems to be developmentally disabled. Maynard points out that as soon as the doctor attaches a linguistic label to what he perceives to be wrong with the child, the child's difficulty becomes a fact, which raises a problem if the parents resist the labeling. Giving labels is also an activity negotiated during talk, and it becomes the starting point for further interaction:

> Stated differently, that a person has a problem can become a taken-for-granted or presumed feature of interaction between clinician and parent so that they can then negotiate specific diagnoses or labels. Such a presumed feature is no automatic, cognitive "seeing and saying" process that participants share, but rather a methodic accomplishment that resides in discourse practices such as those of making and accepting problem proposals within an organized sequence for the delivery of diagnostic news. (Maynard 1988:319–20)

In the context of domestic violence victims doctors' labeling becomes problematic if the labels convey a picture of the woman as incompetent. As Loseke and Cahill (1984) show in their study on the social construction of notions of deviance, experts on battered women such as academic researchers, social service providers, journalists, and political activists have created a new category of deviance by defining victims of domestic violence in a deeply discrediting manner, presenting them largely as women who are unable to manage their own affairs. This ultimately leads to an indirect form of victimization: "As a result, the experts on battered women have constructed a situation where victims of wife assault may lose control over their self-definitions, interpretations of experience, and, in some cases, control over their private affairs. In a sense, battered women may now be victimized twice, first by their mates and then by the experts who claim to speak on their behalf" (Loseke and Cahill 1984:306). It is therefore important to look closely at the way GPs label and define domestic violence, and one objective of this study is to find out whether the GPs' discourse reveals indirect victimization on the linguistic level.

Hunter (1991) draws an analogy between doctor-patient interaction and reading by contending that, in a sense, doctors "read the patient as text." They match the symptoms with well-known patterns of illness and finally create their own narratives of what they have diagnosed and of how they arrived at their conclusion:

> Medicine is practised by means of a series of narrative accounts of illness told in a relatively self-enclosed dialect and according to strict rules that define the genre. These stories or case histories are themselves readings and interpretations of events as they have been represented in patients' narratives or as they have left marks on patients' bodies. . . . Physicians are the readers of these texts, and, like all readers, they read by understanding the signs and fitting them together into a recognizable, communicable whole. (Hunter 1991:8)

Fitting the patient's story into "a recognizable, communicable whole" refers to the ways in which patients' narratives are recoded in a very specialized and powerful language that manifests itself in GPs' notes and case reports. Doctors "rewrite" the patient's original narrative of what he or she thought might be wrong. This process comes close to what Fairclough terms "rewording": "An existing, dominant, and naturalized, wording is being systematically replaced by another one in conscious opposition to it" (1989:113).

In her study on protective order interviews with Latina survivors of domestic abuse, Trinch (2001a, 2001b, 2003) demonstrates how the requirements of writing a protective order application in a district attorney's office and in a pro bono law clinic lead to the "rewriting" of the victims' narratives as reports and even hinder narrative production during the interviews: "In both settings, narrative trajectories are at best negotiated between clients and interviewers and at worst, interviewers impose them. In this regard, both paid paralegals and volunteers act as gatekeepers. Rather than giving clients a chance to narrate freely and represent abuse according to their own narrative practices, both sets of interviewers elicit from clients what it is that they believe is needed to obtain an order" (2001a:496). Thus, Trinch argues, victims may feel unaccompanied in the sociolegal system, and, as a consequence of the interviewers' gatekeeping function, they may "perceive a 'second assault' by the institutions meant to serve them" (2001a:475). Lawless (2001) makes similar observations about the discrepancy between the stories women tell when they seek refuge in shelters and the "official" narratives that are required in police investigations or court proceedings, for example. She contends that institutional rewordings of abused women's narratives in fact deprive these women of their trust in the validity of their own narratives and thereby also impoverish otherwise powerful testimonies of violence: "We teach them to disbelieve and to dishonour their own words and stories by the ways in which the institutions that are supposedly in place for their assistance seek to reshape their words and rewrite their stories to fit the discourse of the service organizations and the courts of law" (Lawless 2001:41–42). What is needed, Lawless argues, is an acknowledgment of "the power of narrative with which we speak ourselves into being" (2001:159).

If victims of domestic violence were given more opportunities to "speak themselves into being" during a consultation and to disclose the violence they suffer, many of the problems general practice currently has with dealing with this issue could be solved (see chapters 3 and 4). After all, a collection of cases or, better, "stories" about cases becomes the knowledge base GPs can draw upon over the years: "Physicians acquire a collection of cases that they have either treated themselves or observed directly, and they augment these with others reported in journals. . . . [T]his practical knowledge informs the interpretation of each new case as the clinician goes about fitting it to the clinical taxonomy of diagnosis and therapy" (Hunter 1991:44–45). Moreover, the cases doctors remember also give them indirect guidelines as to what to look out for the next time a patient comes in with similar symptoms. Narratives consequently form a crucial element in medicine, especially where the symptoms presented by the patient do not match the biomedical model alone.

A lot of the illnesses doctors encounter nowadays have a psychosocial dimension to them and run the risk of remaining undiscovered or underestimated within a "hard science" paradigm in medical practice. As Hunter repeatedly emphasizes in her book, medicine is not, strictly speaking, a science but "a rational, science-using, inter-level, interpretive activity" (1990:25). This insight has gradually made its way into medical theory and has informed a number of studies on the relationship between narrative and medicine, as can be seen in a collection of articles entitled *Narrative Based Medicine* (Greenhalgh and Hurwitz 1998). This collection is mainly addressed to health care professionals and aims at raising awareness about the importance of language in medical encounters. Elwyn and Gwyn, for example, conclude their article on doctor-patient discourse in consultations by stating that "by being aware of certain signalling practices and discourse markers in the patient's talk, general practitioners might be able to listen more constructively to their patients' stories" (1998:174). Ironically, research on doctor-patient communication and on the problems arising from it has a long tradition in sociolinguistics (Shuy 1976; Cicourel 1981; Fisher and Todd 1983; West 1984; Tannen and Wallat 1986) and in the sociology of health and illness (Bennett 1976; Mishler 1984; Silverman 1987). The fact that these findings have only recently started to be taken more seriously in medical practice shows the lack of communication amongst disciplines in the past, communication that could have proved useful a lot earlier for all disciplines involved.

It is not only the patients' narratives, however, that should be given more attention. Patients' narratives have been addressed so assiduously as to imply that physicians do not have any. While GPs are assumed to be the custodians of expert knowledge expressed in a scientific discourse, patients are taken as possessors of folk beliefs expressed in vernacular stories. It is not only important to reintroduce narrative in professional communication and to make the narrative mode acceptable even in "scientific" areas (Perkins and Blyler 1999), but the narrative practices that are already in place in professions such as health care also need to come under closer scrutiny. My narrative angle of entry illuminates something different from the expert knowledge typically attributed to medical professionals. It reveals that physicians are also a folk group with narrative traditions and private lore.

After all, doctors' stories about domestic violence also reflect GPs' participation in a certain "community of practice," that is, "an aggregate of people who come together around mutual engagement in an endeavour. Ways of doing things, ways of talking, beliefs, values, power relations—in short, practice—emerge in the course of this mutual endeavour" (Eckert and McConnell-Ginet 1992:464). This means that GPs share, for example, the sources of their case-based knowledge to the extent that they read the same journal articles and discuss problematic cases with each other. Moreover, GPs, like people from other walks of life, often engage in conversations with each other outside

their professional domain because they have become close friends, for example, or because they pursue the same hobbies. Doctors tell stories to other doctors. It is by virtue of these in-group tellings that folklore can become "storied
knowledge." Furthermore, GPs are not only members of a professional group,
but they are also part of a larger social institution: the health care sector. We
can therefore ask, Are there signs of a common knowledge base and a code of
practice that GPs both draw upon and also re-create and reinforce during the interviews? Is it possible to sift a common narrative out of all the individual narratives that indicates that GPs' linguistic behavior is informed by their professional "community of practice"? As Linde points out, "narratives in groups and
institutions are not solely individual productions, but rather are constrained
by the narratives that have a long-term life within the institution, as well as by
the practices and occasions on which narrative [*sic*] are told" (1997b:286). The
sum of narratives that are related to (re)produce the identity and culture of institutions in bureaucratic settings forms what Linde calls "institutional memory," and narrative also functions "to project the future, in constructing a record that can serve as an institutional memory available in case of possible
challenges" (1999:139).[8]

The concept of institutional memory is not static, as Trinch (2001b) argues,
since it allows for novel narratives that may gradually change an existing institutional memory.[9] Trinch further contends that institutional memory can also
be deficient, as it is "only as complete as the interactions that go into the narrative stories and reports that produce it" (2001b:579).[10] Do doctors also have "institutionalized" narratives about domestic violence, and if so, how accurately
do they reflect women's manifold and complex experiences of violence? If the
GPs' narratives analyzed in this study prove to be very similar in both their content and their linguistic presentation, we can infer that the doctors' discourse
has not only been influenced by the linguistic community of practice in which
the GPs participate but also that their shared notions about domestic violence
incorporated in their "institutional memory" have established a social reality surrounding the issue of domestic violence that GPs take for a fact. Following from there, a case can be made for sociolinguistic analysis as a crucial tool
in investigating the relationship between structural linguistic units and social
practices (Linde 1997a). This seems to be particularly relevant in the context of

present-day society, "where the public life of society members is materially affected by public agencies" (Gumperz and Cook-Gumperz 1982:4).

In this study primary health care as part of the larger medical sector and thus by default also as a social institution comes under closer scrutiny. I demonstrate to what extent GPs' narrative constructions of domestic violence as a social problem reveal and at the same time underpin professional practices that might have an impact on the relevant service provision women suffering domestic abuse may or may not receive when they go to see their family doctor. A number of studies have analyzed the community response to violence (Eekelaar and Katz 1978; Borkowski, Murch, and Walker 1983; Pahl 1985; Tayside Women and Violence Group 1994), including legal, medical, and social services. Other studies have concentrated on individual areas such as the criminal justice system and criminology (Stanko 1985, 1990), social work (Dobash, Dobash, and Cavanagh 1985; Lloyd 1995), and the response to domestic violence in psychiatric and medical emergency departments (Bograd 1987; Warshaw 1993; Campbell et al. 1994; Keller 1996; Pahl 1995). More recently, studies have also taken into account general practice as one setting where domestic abuse is disclosed (Bradley et al. 2002; Richardson et al. 2002). Despite the diverse characteristics of these institutions, the results are strikingly similar in that they portray a relatively gloomy picture as far as the service provision for victims of domestic abuse is concerned.[11] One aim of this book is to uncover, by means of narrative analysis, possible problems underlying doctor-patient interaction with regard to domestic abuse. For example, do the GPs' narratives and their linguistic features offer any explanation for the lack of consistent service provision? I take a closer look at domestic violence and general practice in the next chapter.

3. Domestic Violence and the Role of General Practice
A Narrative-Analytic Approach

Cohen (1992) shows that women have sought shelter and, at the same time, have been institutionalized for a wide array of reasons ever since the Middle Ages, including protection and assistance but also punishment and rehabilitation. In the past institutions for women were mainly run by the church, and their diverse functions presented a double-edged sword: on the one hand, women were offered material help and refuge in their socioeconomic plights; on the other hand, clerical institutions also saw it as their task to "reform" prostitutes and equally "deviant" women (Cohen 1992:169). This example demonstrates that violence against women has had a long history and that, moreover, it has largely been condoned by society. At the same time, the boundaries between domestic and institutional violence are shown to be far from clear-cut. Despite its long history and prevalence in our society, domestic violence only became topical as part of a more general feminist resistance to patriarchal structures and male dominance in the late 1960s and came to be perceived as a political issue in the early seventies, when the battered women's movement started to emerge in Britain under the auspices of Erin Pizzey and her associates (Johnson 1995:102–4). The first British community center for women and their children was set up in 1972 under the name of Chiswick Women's Aid, which received extensive media coverage, and from there information as well as practical help were offered throughout the country.

The emergence of Women's Aid groups and the politicization of domestic violence were accompanied by growing research interest in domestic violence, particularly its various forms, causes, and consequences (Steinmetz and Straus 1974; Gelles 1976; Eekelaar and Katz 1978; Dobash and Dobash 1979).[1] Since researchers in preceding decades had hardly addressed the issue, one major concern in the seventies was to find out the extent of domestic violence. As a consequence, quantitative studies and survey research abound in the literature of the time. These data were closely linked with researchers' attempts to generate theories of family violence. Gelles identifies three main explanatory models in the seventies within which theories of violence were formulated: (1) the "psychiatric model," which focuses on the perpetrator's personality and related factors such as mental illness and alcohol or drug abuse; (2) the "social-psychological model," which examines external environmental factors such as stresses, family histories of violence over generations, and family interaction patterns; and (3) the "sociocultural model," which takes into account macrolevel structures of inequality, cultural attitudes, and norms (1980:881). These explanatory models have partly survived and still constitute frameworks for investigation. Willson et al. (2000) and Johnson (2001), for example, analyze the correlations between alcohol or drug abuse and violence against women by intimate partners. Although Willson et al. identify a correlation between alcohol or drug abuse and intensity of violence, both Willson et al. and Johnson caution against the oversimplified view that there is a causal connection. Johnson in particular concludes from her data that "male attitudes and beliefs in the rightness of control over female partners made a more important statistical contribution than did alcohol, age, type of relationship, or class variables. The acting-out of negative attitudes toward women, especially men's rights to degrade and devalue their female partners through name-calling and putdowns, was an especially important predictor and, once entered, reduced the effects of alcohol abuse to nonsignificance" (2001:68). Feminist researchers have also challenged the attribution of intimate partner violence to external stress factors such as low income, unemployment, and so on as well as cycle-of-abuse theories and transmission of violence over generations. Such explanations are problematic, since "in a variety of ways, violence is socially legitimated" (Johnson 1995:116). Johnson continues by arguing that "while stress resulting from poverty, inequality and various forms of deprivation may be contributory factors in domestic violence, only a small proportion of those who experience such conditions behave violently towards their partners, and many of those who do behave violently are neither poor nor deprived" (1995:116). This raises questions concerning the generation and interpretation of survey figures in studies operating within the social-psychological framework. In their review of data from the first National Family Violence Survey conducted in America by Straus, Gelles, and Steinmetz, Johnson and Ferraro (2000) show, for example, that the effects stated in cycle-of-violence theories are in fact small. While Straus, Gelles, and Steinmetz claimed that the wife-beating rate for sons of violent parents was 1,000 percent greater than that of sons of nonviolent parents, Johnson and Ferraro reinterpret the actual rate of 20 percent as "meaning that even among this group of men whose parents were two standard deviations above average in level of partner violence, 80% of the adult sons had not even once in the last 12 months committed any acts of severe violence toward their partners" (2000:958). In other words, the fact that some men witness violence as children does not necessarily mean that they become abusive themselves. Williamson argues along the same lines by stating that "without more consistent and thorough evidence, cycle of abuse theories cannot be utilised as an adequate explanation for the occurrence of domestic violence, as they do not explain why men who also experience domestic violence as children do not go on to abuse their own partners" (2000:95).

Most researchers nowadays agree that domestic violence is not tied to any specific sociodemographic factor but that it occurs across all social classes, cultural and ethnic backgrounds, and age groups. However, differences may exist in terms of types and presentations of abuse, which requires further differentiation and attention to subtle details, as Johnson and Ferraro (2000:959) postulate. I would argue that it is equally important to consider the wider social context in which violence is made possible and the influential role of social institutions and their discursive practices in the process of victimization.

The violence women experience takes many forms and covers a wide range of abusive behavior that can be subsumed under at least three categories: physical violence, emotional abuse, and sexual abuse (Mazza, Dennerstein, and Ryan 1996:15). In addition, Gay (1997) investigates "linguistic violence" as a special form of violence. Violent men beat, cut, and burn their partners, they break their bones and teeth, they tear out their hair, and they rape them. It is not surprising that general practitioners are often the first person to see and witness the results of abuse (Scottish Needs Assessment Programme 1997). Furthermore, the often prolonged duration of abusive relationships and the severity of violent attacks some women are exposed to often lead to chronic illness and a range of emotional and psychiatric problems such as depression, anxiety, post-traumatic stress disorder (PTSD), and suicide (British Medical Association 1998:30; Campbell 2002). For these reasons the Department of Health highlights right at the beginning of its resource manual for health care professionals the unique role health services potentially fulfill: "Health services have a pivotal role to play in the identification, assessment and response to domestic violence, not only because of the impact of domestic violence on health, but crucially because the health services may often be the only contact point with professionals who could recognise and intervene in the situation" (2000:2).[2] All that is said here about medical services in general also applies to GPs, who often have an even closer relationship with patients in their role as family doctor. As Annandale (1998:143–44) points out, women from around the age of ten to the midsixties are much more likely to consult their GP than men. And yet studies have shown that doctors and other medical staff do not always detect domestic violence in their patients.[3] This raises a number of questions concerning the disclosure and detection of domestic violence in general practice. Do GPs really encounter only a few patients who suffer domestic violence, or do they overlook possible cases? If they do not detect domestic violence, is it because women do not open up or because GPs are reluctant to broach the subject? Are they not sensitized enough to possible underlying issues? If this is the case, what could be the reasons? Abbott and Williamson locate the problem in GPs' "failure" to find out about domestic violence: "These figures suggest that health care professionals significantly underestimate the extent of domestic violence and are failing to 'detect' it as the cause of injuries and other health problems reported by their female patients" (1999:91). It is also a fact, however, that women often need a long time before they disclose their problem to their GP. Henderson (1997) points out that some patients return to their doctor's office up to thirty times before managing to disclose domestic violence. A prevalence survey conducted in Melbourne by Mazza, Dennerstein, and Ryan (1996) showed that only 27 percent of the women who had experienced partner or childhood physical abuse had actually disclosed this to their doctor. The main reason respondents offered for not communicating their problem to their doctor was "not because they were afraid, embarrassed or untrusting, but because they were never asked" (Mazza, Dennerstein, and Ryan 1996:16).

Why do women not disclose and doctors not ask? Dobash and Dobash talk about a "conspiracy of silence" (1979:181) between doctor and patient, that is, a mutual denial of the violence at stake where women fabricate explanations for injuries and doctors accept them without further inquiry. Studies have shown that women often deny violence because of shame, fear of retaliation, and continued trauma (Dobash and Dobash 1979:180) but also because they sense a lack of advocacy and interest from their GP (Williamson 2000:47–65). An ethno-graphic study by Sugg and Inui (1992), who are also medical doctors, yielded a number of interesting results concerning doctors' reluctance to ask about domestic violence. First, doctors stated a close identification with patients of the same socioeconomic background. This entails two consequences: on the one hand, patients from a higher social background are less likely to be identified as victims of abuse because they are not asked; on the other hand, the misconception of domestic violence as a product of poverty is perpetuated through the selective questioning of patients from lower social classes (Sugg and Inui 1992:3160). Another issue raised by physicians was their fear of offending the patient, which Sugg and Inui regard as stemming from cultural constructs of what is private. In other words, doctors do not think they are in a position to interfere in patients' private matters, and domestic violence is regarded as a private matter. A third concern was related to doctors' feeling of powerlessness and a sense of inadequacy, as medical tools were regarded as inappropriate. This argument was closely linked to a fourth problem, namely, the GPs' frustration with their lack of power in a situation in which they could not control whether a patient accepted and followed their advice. However, the most pervasive and driving fear expressed by the doctors was the time factor. Time pressure is likely to prevent a physician from delving into a problem that is potentially offensive or difficult to resolve. As I show in my analyses, these explanations are constantly recycled in GPs' narrative discourse and thus preclude a paradigm shift at the level of GPs' "storied knowledge" of the problem.

The severe lack of communication between GPs and patients who experience domestic violence has far-reaching consequences and huge implications for primary care in terms of morbidity, GPs' workload, and long-term costs.[4] It is not least on these grounds that primary care ought to be seen as a key setting for further exploration. More important, however, I would argue with Williamson that "healthcare professionals have a moral imperative to deal with the issue of domestic violence as social citizens, in conjunction with their professional responsibility" (2000:59). Even though GPs cannot treat the causes, prevent the effects, or assure the cures for men hurting women, they are gatekeepers to whom women might disclose because their injuries precipitate narratives of how the injuries were sustained. As I mentioned above, women have periodic, intimate, and physical contact with GPs that might serve as an occasion of disclosure even if there are no physical symptoms. In my view GPs have a moral obligation to at least keep the gate open and facilitate disclosure.

The Biomedical Model and the "Appropriation of the Sick Role"

In order to understand the difficulties GPs might have in dealing with cases of domestic violence it is important to clarify the concept of the biomedical model of medicine first, since this is the model upon which most of today's mainstream medical practice is based. The history of medicine and of conceptual models used in medical practice was highly influenced by two major developments: first, the rise of the hospital as a medical institution, initially in France in the early nineteenth century (Foucault 1973); and second, the emergence of "laboratory medicine" in the mid-nineteenth century, that is, medicine that was informed by increasing scientific knowledge of physiochemical processes (Annandale 1998). Thus the "birth" of modern medicine, to draw upon Foucault's metaphor, can be located in the wider context of the industrial revolution, with its dynamic processes of industrialization, the movement of the population from the countryside into the cities, and the rise of capitalism. While up until the eighteenth century medical practitioners worked within a "person-oriented cosmology" (Annandale 1998:5), in which judgments were made by taking into account the patient's personality as a whole, the patient gradually disappeared into the mass of hospital patients waiting for treatment. What is more, since the rise of the hospital provided doctors with greater financial autonomy, doctor-patient relationships were no longer based on good rapport and negotiation of interpretations of illness, and the control over medical knowledge was entirely passed from the patient to the doctor. This development was of course supported by doctors' increasingly specialized knowledge in the area of biomedicine. The patient, on the other hand, was almost reduced to a material entity to be analyzed. As Annandale puts it, in "the eighteenth century the sick person was conceived as a 'whole person'; today the body is typically viewed as a complex machine apart from the mind" (1998:6).

In line with the biomedical model doctors treat whatever is physically wrong with the patient, but they do not judge the patient on personal or moral grounds. In a way, doctors are claimed to be "clinical" in every sense of the word. As O'Connor remarks: "In keeping with the scientific tradition, modern biomedicine has striven to separate itself from broader cultural concerns and influences"

(1995:22). When it comes to identifying and treating medical problems that do not match the biomedical model alone but that have psychosocial origins, however, these assumptions obviously pose difficulties. In the case of domestic violence abuse cannot, strictly speaking, be viewed as an illness and thus does not fall within the duties and responsibilities of medicine. Furthermore, since the causes of abuse are not definable within a biophysical framework, GPs may find it puzzling to identify their own role as suitable to deal with this problem.

Another factor in this context is what Williamson (2000) calls the "appropriation of the sick role," that is, the process whereby patients' illnesses are legitimized by the doctor. As Williamson points out, the "sick role" encompasses a number of components:

> First, the sick role legitimates abdication of social responsibility for the duration of the illness. Second, the abdication of social and familial responsibilities is dependent on the seeking of professional help and advice. Third, the individual is responsible for assisting in the recovery process, through adherence to the professional recommendations they receive. Finally, there is an expectation that individuals seek help from specifically trained, and therefore legitimated, health providers. (2000:19)

All these components instantiate the social control function of doctors and of medical discourse: a patient is considered "genuinely ill" only if his or her illness is defined as such by the doctor. The appropriation of the sick role has, of course, implications for victims of domestic violence. What do general practitioners regard as "illness" or "disease" in medical terms? What do they assume concerning the level of responsibility and agency women attain in domestic violence situations? Doctors may well assume that women are partly responsible for the violence they experience and therefore consider resulting injuries as almost self-inflicted. Similarly, if women do not follow doctors' advice to leave an abusive partner, this might be viewed as a breach of the rules pertaining to the sick role. As a consequence, doctors may distinguish between "legitimate" and "illegitimate" states of health and illness, which deserve different levels of treatment. This differentiation in turn can lead to the stigmatization of the patient's behavior as inappropriate (Williamson 2000:20).

Cultural Myths and Explanatory Frameworks

Keller proposes psychological explanations for the problem and sees the evaluation of a battered woman as a "crisis setting" (1996:8) that can lead to psychological pressure on service providers. Countertransference mechanisms can then cause misguided projections of anger, sadness, or anxiety onto the patient and thus prove detrimental for treatment or therapy. Bograd analyzes clinical approaches to battered women from a feminist perspective and reaches the conclusion that they are "based less on scientific formulation and research than on prevailing male-defined cultural myths about women" (1987:69). Williamson (2000) also reveals GPs' reluctance to tackle the problem and uncovers some of the misconceptions and stigmatizing clichés GPs succumb to and, at the same time, reinforce in their discourses about patients. What are these myths? Since I also use the term *cultural myths* when referring to some of the GPs' conceptualizations, I provide an overview at this point to make the framework for this study more transparent to readers.

In line with Schornstein (1997:24–30), who surveyed a great range of empirical studies on domestic violence and to whom I would like to refer the interested reader, I take the following twelve assumptions to be myths about causes for and dynamics of domestic violence:

1. *Myth*: The victim caused the violence. She "asked for it."
   Fact: The batterer caused the violence. He is responsible for his actions.

2. *Myth*: The victim enjoys the abuse. If she didn't enjoy it, she would leave him.
   Fact: No one enjoys being beaten.

3. *Myth*: Domestic violence is a family or private matter.
   Fact: Domestic violence is a crime against the victim and against society.

4. *Myth*: If the victim left the batterer, the violence would stop.
   Fact: Most victims are in greater danger of increased violence after they leave the abuser.

5. *Myth*: Alcohol and drug abuse cause domestic violence.
   Fact: Generally speaking, alcohol and drug use do not cause violent behavior.

6. *Myth*: Domestic violence only occurs in lower socioeconomic groups.
   Fact: Domestic violence occurs in all socioeconomic groups.
7. *Myth*: The incidence of domestic violence is overstated. It is not that much of a problem.
   Fact: Domestic violence is a significant problem for women all over the world.
8. *Myth*: Women are just as violent as men.
   Fact: Men make up the overwhelming percentage of domestic violence perpetrators.
9. *Myth*: Battered women gravitate to abusers. Even if such women leave their violent partners, they will just find other men who will beat them.
   Fact: Women do not seek abusive partners.
10. *Myth*: The assault is an isolated incident, unlikely to happen again.
    Fact: Battering is part of a complex pattern of domination and control.
11. *Myth*: Domestic violence is merely "a push and a shove."
    Fact: Batterers engage in countless forms of violence.
12. *Myth*: If he beat her up, he must be mentally ill.
    Fact: Mental illness is not a prerequisite for domestic violence.

I consider domestic violence a complex and multifactorial problem that is also culturally constructed and "made sense of" by means of discursive practices. Williamson (2000) too emphasizes the significance of doctors' *discourse* in her study, and yet her discussion of interview excerpts remains largely a content analysis. So how is domestic violence linguistically constructed? How can a narrative-analytic approach yield insights into the construction of cultural and institutional narratives about domestic violence? Before I move on to a discussion of the narrative frame model for my study I briefly present my research methodology and the data used for the analyses.

Research Methodology
The twenty in-depth interviews for this study were conducted in the city of Aberdeen between March and July 2000. Aberdeen is a cosmopolitan port in

northeastern Scotland. Compared to other countries such as Finland and Sweden, for example, Scotland takes a national partnership approach toward domestic violence based on gendered notions of the problem (McKie 2004). The Partnership Strategy (Scottish Executive 2000), which followed the advent of the first Scottish Parliament in three hundred years in 1999, initiated multiagency partnerships and required local authorities to devise action plans and strategies. Reviewed legislation enhanced the protection of women. Thus, the Protection from Abuse(s) Act came into force in 2001, and the Criminal Justice Bill and the Sexual Offences Act 2002 reinforced protection, particularly from sexual offenses. In other words, I conducted this study at a time when the problem of domestic abuse was prominent in public debates and therefore also had some media coverage.

The respondents for this study were selected by means of purposive sampling from a list of doctors' office addresses issued by the Grampian NHS Board.[5] Purposive sampling involves respondents' selection according to certain preestablished criteria (Mason 1996:94). The criteria for this study were (1) an equal split of male and female GPs in the sample and (2) practices from a wide geographical catchment area comprising both city center and suburban areas of Aberdeen. The aim was to have a variety of practices with patients from different socioeconomic backgrounds in order to test the assumption that this may influence doctors' experiences with domestic violence.[6] It was difficult to control the sample for the age variable, since information on age is not easily available. Other difficulties included problems of access and nonresponse. Thus when I phoned up to arrange an interview it required patience and insistence to pass by receptionists in order to speak to the GPs themselves. Receptionists obviously fulfill a gatekeeping function in medical practices. Their task is to ward off all "unwanted" calls or callers asking for the GP's time who are not patients. Eventually, out of the fifty-five GPs I wrote to, thirty-seven declined to be interviewed. Most of them mentioned lack of time as the main reason for why they could not participate. A few GPs stated that they did not think domestic violence was an issue for them.

Nevertheless, the sample finally included GPs from a fairly wide age range and, more important, a wide range of years of experience in general practice, with some GPs being at the beginning of their careers and others nearing retirement. The range was between three and thirty-three years of general practice work. The sample of twenty GPs consisted of eleven male and nine female doctors from sixteen different practices, three of which were situated in the city center, eleven in the wider city area, three on the outskirts of the city, and three in suburbs to the north, northwest, and southwest of Aberdeen. The fact that eight of the doctors in my sample worked in joint practices and thus held office hours in at least two different parts of town throughout the week allowed for an even wider catchment area to be covered. Whether the practice was situated in an affluent, upper-middle-class area or in a deprived area in town did not seem to matter too much in the interviews because many GPs were able to draw on experiences they had had elsewhere, in other practices, in other cities, even in other countries.

The interview schedule was semistructured and considerably loose. The questions I asked were phrased freely around the following catchwords, which had emerged from previous pilot interviews: time; silence; emotions when dealing with patients; definition of domestic violence; experiences; reasons for domestic violence; problem of opening up; reluctance to broach the subject; relevance in general practice; status of domestic violence in the health care system in general; consultation; signs/signals of domestic violence; action/steps to be taken; range of services available to women; training. The length of the interviews ranged between fourteen and thirty-seven minutes due to the GPs' concerns about their lack of time, with most of the interviews lasting for approximately half an hour. All the interviews were taped and transcribed. The transcription conventions used for this study (see also "Transcription Conventions") are adopted, with minor changes, from Norrick (2000). The overall aim was to leave the interview text as readable and accessible as possible.[7] Thus, an analysis of metaphoric language or of passive constructions does not necessarily require a close phonetic transcription, for example, while an investigation into turn taking, back channels, and other interactional features demands a minimum notation of pauses and intonational patterns (e.g., stress).

The Corpus
In sum, thirty-six narratives could be extracted from the interviews (see appendix). Narratives were identified by the following criteria for a prototypical story: "A prototypical story identifies a protagonist, a predicament, attempts to resolve the predicament, the outcomes of such attempts, and the reactions of

the protagonists to the situation. Causal relationships among each of the story elements are also explicitly identified in the prototype" (Robinson and Hawpe 1986:112). In other words, passages in the interviews are considered narratives if they depart from GPS' general accounts and discussions of domestic violence and introduce a personal story that incorporates some or all of the above criteria. Not all narratives in my data match the "prototype" entirely. Thus a few narratives were only initiated but not related in full length. Other narratives appeared fragmented throughout the interview, for example, when doctors referred back to a case they had mentioned earlier or when I prompted them to tell me more about a case. In these instances narratives were identified and counted but not necessarily included in the analysis because they did not lend themselves to the narrative approach as it is adopted here.

Another reason why I did not take some of the narratives into account is the fact that they are only marginally related to the issue of domestic violence. One narrative, for example, depicts a case of child sexual abuse, and another one discusses the practice work of a GP's former colleague. The narratives generated in my sample are of two kinds: twelve were interviewer initiated, that is, they were told in response to questions such as "Can you tell me about your experiences?" and "Is there any case that's particularly vivid in your memory?"; twenty-four narratives, however, can be classified as "spontaneous," as they were told in contexts in which I had not explicitly asked for a story. This underlines the argument put forward in this study and by other authors (Bruner 1986, 1991; Schank 1990; Herman 2002) that narratives are a widely used device in conversation and that they play a crucial role both in the shaping of human understanding and in human interaction. "Storied knowledge" forms a referential framework from which people can retrieve remembered experiences in order to apply them to new or similar situations.

Narrative-Analytic Tools
How can we combine these macrostructural assumptions about narrative and knowledge with the microstructural level of narrative analysis and its narratological tools? The tools for the narrative analysis undertaken in this study are mainly drawn from the sociolinguistic tradition initiated by Labov and Waletzky's (1967) groundbreaking article. Labov and Waletzky and Labov (1982, 1997)

capture the structure of a standard oral narrative in the diamond diagram of narratives. In the *orientation* section the narrator identifies the time, place, persons, and their activity prior to the narrated event or the general situation. The narrative is then developed in a *complicating action* sequence, which leads to a *result* or *resolution*. The narrative can be preceded by an *abstract*, which gives a very brief summary of the following story, and it can be concluded with a *coda*, that is, a general observation or comment made by the narrator to signal that the narrative is finished.

Another key concept is Labov's notion of *temporal juncture*. Two clauses can be said to occur in temporal juncture "if a reversal of their order results in a change in the listener's interpretation of the order of the events described" (Labov 1997:399). Temporal juncture is used by Labov to define a "minimal narrative": "A narrative must contain at least one temporal juncture. . . . Temporal juncture is the simplest, most favored or unmarked way of recounting the past" (1997:399). Narratives can of course take different shapes, for example, through syntactic embedding, use of the past perfect, and so on. In Labov's view these forms are more marked, however. Such markedness is often related to "reportability" in narratives, discussed in greater detail in chapter 9. The assumption is that storytellers usually depict extraordinary or in some ways captivating events in order to justify their telling of the story and to ensure its success in a given situation.

A few caveats need to be added at this point. As I already emphasized above, this study regards narrative as representations of GPs' memorized experience of domestic violence cases and does not aim to present a detailed conversation-analytic approach with close attention to the sequential organization of narrative production. I think that a detailed description of my responses involving mainly back channels such as "mm-hmm" and "yeah" would not really add much to the analyses if it was undertaken for each single narrative, and it would certainly make the narratives tedious to read. For this reason the narratives are mainly treated as products of the interaction between interviewer and GP rather than as sequential interaction as such and are presented accordingly. My choice of line breaks follows Labov and Waletzky's (1967) typology of narrative clauses, which is based on the concept of temporal juncture. The analysis of sequential elements on the narrative context level is restricted to instances where the interactional nature of the interview situation manifests itself in, for example, features expressing politeness, reluctance, self-monitoring, and so on. We must not forget, however, that the distinction between "narrative level" and "narrative context level" is not always as clear-cut. The distinction at best serves as a schematic model. This is nevertheless useful, I think, as it brings into sharper relief factors influencing narrative production.

A Frame Model for Interview Narratives

In order to understand what is linguistically going on in the interviews with the GPs and hence in their narratives it helps to consider the interview situation at large. An analytical model of oral narratives needs to take into account at least the medium, spatiotemporal contexts, the role of the participants, and the purpose or function of a narrative in any given situation. Schiffrin (1993), for example, shows in her study on the phenomenon "talking for another" that the interview situation sets a dominant frame to which participants accommodate their speech but at the same time apply strategies of "in-frame" and "out-of-frame" conversation, that is, conversation that either remains within the expectational boundaries of the interview frame (e.g., the question-answer pattern) or goes beyond it. Any linguistic interaction can be interpreted in terms of frames of expectations and socially codified rules, as Tannen (1993b) points out. Frame theory goes back to the work of Erving Goffman, who conceptualized conversation as a staged play during which participants act out their roles as individuals but also as social and professional personae: "Often what talkers undertake to do is not to provide information to a recipient but to present dramas to an audience. Indeed, it seems that we spend most of our time not engaged in giving information but in giving shows" (1974:509). The term *frame* includes organizational rules for interaction on both social as well as personal levels. Thus, Goffman assumes that "definitions of a situation are built up in accordance with principles of organization which govern events—at least social ones—and our subjective involvement in them" (1974:10–11). Goffman labels the sum of these basic principles underlying a given situation as a "frame."

I adopt Goffman's concept of frame in order to depict the contextual frames relevant to my study. The schematic model in figure 1 captures the embeddedness of interview narratives within these larger conceptual and interactional frames. The interview narrative forms the nucleus of a first interactional frame, the narrative frame. Narratives, and with them the narrative frame, are optional elements inside the interview frame; that is, they occur as one of several discursive

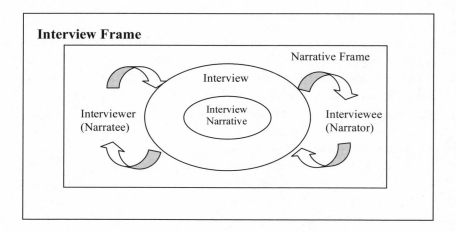

devices the interviewee can but need not necessarily draw upon. One interview script in my sample does not contain any narrative, for example. The narrative frame is embedded in a larger contextual frame, namely, the interview frame. Let me provide an overview of the different frames and what they entail.

The Narrative Frame

Within the narrative frame the storyteller relates a "story" to the listener. Since the listener, or "narratee," however, brings certain culturally and socially defined expectations to bear upon the narrative frame (e.g., judgments as to what a "good" narrative should be like and whether it is relevant in the particular conversational situation) and since to some extent the storyteller accommodates his or her narrative to these expectations, it is more appropriate to talk about a "co-construction," or a jointly created narrative. Gumperz distinguishes two types of inferences speakers make in conversation: "First, there are those inferences that retrieve background knowledge on what the frame or activity is. That is, knowledge that suggests what the interaction involves, what the appropriate relationships among interactants are, and what outcomes are expected. Secondly, there are the inferences that enter into what we may call conversational management, such as the allocation of turns at speaking, the maintenance of thematic cohesion and the signaling of topic change" (1997:195). Gumperz clearly favors a conversation-analytic approach that is founded on detailed analysis of the sequential organization of talk. In the context of interview narratives, however, a close sequential analysis is not always useful, since the interviewer's turns are mostly marked by back channels such as "mm-hmm," "yeah," and so on, which are normally used as fairly neutral interaction devices to encourage the interviewee to hold the floor. Moreover, as I mentioned above, narratives can be regarded as products of speakers' memorized stock of narrative knowledge and can therefore be analyzed holistically. Nevertheless, an in-depth analysis of the narrative frame has to take into account not only the structural details of the narrative proper, or what I would like to label "narrative features," but also assumptions about exactly those expectations and norms that inform "online" narrative construction and all aspects surrounding the narrative, its "narrative context features." These features include not only linguistic cues and aspects but also gaze, gestures, and body language.

"Interview talk" should never be confused with "natural speech," as Wolfson (1976) emphasizes. Interview talk is not "natural," as it is always influenced by speakers' consciousness of the presence of the tape recorder. Labov calls this phenomenon the "observer's paradox" (i.e., the observer tries "to find out how people talk when they are not being systematically observed" [1972b:209], and the only way to obtain these data is by systematic observation). During the interviews the observer's paradox was noticeable in the way some of the GPs repeatedly glanced at the dictaphone. One GP openly stated after the interview that the presence of the dictaphone had been "intimidating." The presence of the tape recorder certainly has to account for omissions in the doctors' stories and for self-monitoring mechanisms, which could be seen in statements such as "I'm not gonna make defensive answers." As a consequence of the observer's paradox, interview narratives are not introduced in a natural manner and solely on the interview subject's initiative. Instead, they are often direct responses to interview questions or prompts and therefore appear more like summaries: "The conversational narrative is related to and inspired by the topic under discussion. Changes in topic are usually motivated by something within the conversation. In contrast, the question/answer rule of the interview prevents the speaker from introducing topics of narratives" (Wolfson 1976:192). Wolfson makes a valid point. The narrative data generated in my interviews with the GPs would look different had they been derived from private conversations between doctors and their spouses or partners, doctors and their colleagues, or even doctors and their patients. I am not saying that those conversations would be more "natural," but they would certainly be less formal and would follow different rules and principles.

We could object here that doctor-patient communication is also very formal and highly regulated. This is true; and yet, from a GP's point of view, the whole situation would probably be regarded more as a professional routine in which a doctor simply acts out his or her more or less predetermined role (Young 1997:16), while in an interview the fact that another person asks questions and that the interview is being taped can be quite intimidating. The main difference, I think, lies in the power dynamics between the conversational partners in these two speech situations. As Marková and Foppa point out, any dialogue contains asymmetry as a built-in feature:

> While dialogues must, by definition, be reciprocal, interlocutors differ in their control of the content, quality and quantity of their dialogical contributions and, consequently, equality or symmetricity between them is exceptional. . . . As interlocutors set and take perspectives, mutually construct the meaning of what they say, develop intersubjective relationships and impart knowledge, they reduce certain dialogical asymmetries while establishing others. In this sense asymmetries are inherent in the dynamics of dialogue. (1991:259–60)

The interview situation becomes even more asymmetrical when interviews are conducted with professionals. Strangely enough, the asymmetry works in two ways: on the one hand, there is an axis going from the interviewer to the interviewee, with the interviewer as the person who asks questions being in a more powerful position; on the other hand, another axis runs diametrically opposed to the first one from the GP to the interviewer because now the focus is on the GP as an expert in his or her field from whom the researcher wishes to gain information. This in itself is already an interesting point for consideration, since the aim in this study was also to find out how doctors as *professionals* react linguistically to a topic such as domestic violence.

The Interview Frame

As indicated in the model, listener and storyteller take up their roles as interviewer and interviewee, respectively, in the interview frame. These roles presuppose certain situationally determined behavioral rules and expectations with regard to the organization of turn taking (Sacks, Schegloff, and Jefferson 1974) and the choice of topics to be discussed. As Rubin and Rubin point out, a "normal conversation can drift along with little goal, but in interviews, the re-searcher gently guides the discussion, leading it through stages, asking specific questions, and encouraging the interviewee to answer in depth and at length" (1995:124). Both interviewer and interviewee are of course not merely actors in a more or less clearly demarcated arena, but they also bring into the interview frame the requirements of their social and professional roles and possibly per-sonal and affective characteristics. Another issue is the way interviewer and interviewee perceive each other and how that in turn influences the course of the conversation. In their groundbreaking study on interpersonal perception Laing, Phillipson, and Lee (1966) demonstrate how people's perceptions of each other are in fact the result of complex constructions and reconstructions of self-identities (my view of myself) and meta-identities (my view of your view of me). The interplay of self-identity and meta-identity applies to any human interac-tion, but it comes into sharper relief in an interview, in which interviewer and respondent consciously adopt their respective roles in the interview frame and accommodate their speech and behavior to what they think the other person expects of them. Accommodation theory offers a useful conceptual framework for understanding this process. Interpersonal accommodation theory states that speech style shifts occur among speakers "so as to encourage further interac-tion and decrease the perceived discrepancies between the actors. The assump-tion then is that in such situations, the speaker and the listener have shared a common set of interpretative procedures which allow the speaker's intentions to be (i) encoded by the speaker, and (ii) correctly interpreted by the listener" (Giles and Smith 1979:46–47). In other words, communication is usually based on a common code of practice. Speakers' styles are marked by either "conver-gence" (i.e., "the processes whereby individuals shift their speech styles to be-come more like that of those with whom they are interacting" [Giles and Smith 1979:46]) or "divergence" (i.e., speech "shifts *away* from the interlocutor's style" [Giles and Smith 1979:52]).

The GPs' responses are probably influenced by the fact that they wanted to come across as knowledgeable health care professionals. Equally important are linguistic cues that indicate that the doctors had certain expectations or made assumptions about my expectations of them or what I thought about them as doctors. GPs clearly had the interview frame in mind when they said things like "I'm not being very helpful here" or "My interview is probably flavored by the

fact that I've actually been asked to speak on domestic violence in pregnancies."
Defensive answers, by contrast, might indicate that the GP felt threatened by potential criticism. We must also not forget the sensitive nature of the topic. Since
interpersonal perceptions are crucial determinants of talk-in-interaction, sociodemographic variables such as age, gender, occupation, educational background, and so on have to be identified, if possible, and traced in the dialogues
that emerge between people. More specifically, we can look out for hedges and
boosters as indicators of power dynamics (Holmes 1995), for example, or back
channels, self-corrections, and repairs in turn taking as means of establishing
rapport and of negotiating meaning between interviewer and interviewee.

What is also at stake here is a question of politeness (Lakoff 1977). The interviewee may regard it as potentially impolite behavior to hold the floor for
too long in a conversation. As Sacks, Schegloff, and Jefferson point out, "once
a state of talk has been ratified, cues must be available for requesting the floor
and giving it up, for informing the speaker as to the stability of the focus of attention he is receiving" (1974:697). If a speaker requests the floor for too long,
he or she may appear to be too demanding and ultimately lose the listener's attention. Politeness also plays an important role in interviews, since interviewer
and interviewee meet as strangers who act out specific roles. Researchers may
feel more obliged to behave in a polite manner, since they request the interview-
ees' time and are thus granted a favor.

Another influential factor in social interaction is what Goffman calls "face-
work," that is, "actions taken by a person to make whatever he is doing consistent with face. Face-work serves to counteract 'incidents'—that is, events whose
effective symbolic implications threaten face" (1967:12). In other words, interactants make an effort to save face and to avoid threats to the other person's
face.[8] Goffman assumes that people have an inherent knowledge of the rules required for successful interaction with others, so-called social skills. Thus people know how to evade potentially "face-threatening acts" (FTAs) (Brown and
Levinson 1987). For example, interlocutors remain within the boundaries of the
set expectational frame of a social situation. Taking this as a baseline, we must
approach interview narratives with a view to identifying topics that "are part
of the officially accredited flow" (Goffman 1967:35) and those that go beyond
the interview frame. In my interviews, for example, it is worthwhile exploring
whether the GPs' responses and narratives were given in such a way as to "save"
the GPs' face and to portray them in a specifically positive manner. On the other

hand, we can also look at the strategies GPs applied when they decided to commit a face-threatening act, for example, if they challenged what they perceived as the interviewer's point of view. All this is considered in the analyses of the GPs' narrative discourses in the following chapters. To illustrate the rather theoretical outline of mechanisms of talk-in-interaction with an example, I provide a brief discussion of an interview excerpt here to allow the reader to catch a first glimpse of the data.

Influences of the Interview Frame on Features of Talk-in-Interaction and the Negotiation of Identities

Anticipatory self-criticism occurs relatively frequently across the interviews, albeit to different degrees, and it is indicative of the high level of self-monitoring in the GPs and of the dynamics inherent in the interaction between interviewee and interviewer. It becomes clear from the data that it is extremely difficult to judge in the different instances whether the self-criticism was genuine or whether it was used as a linguistic gesture to create a certain identity of the "good" doctor who knows his or her limitations. Some GPs, by contrast, were quite adamant about not being concerned whether they missed domestic violence cases. The following excerpt shows the interaction between me (the interviewer) and one male middle-aged GP:

> J: Mm-hmm. Do you feel concerned about this, I mean . . . ?
> Dr.: Only when you sit down and think about it. But, er, no [**clears his throat**]. What you do, **you really have got to think what you do,** you've got plenty of other patients as well. **You know,** when you think in terms of each individual patient then **yes,** you're obviously concerned. When you**'ve got** a surgery of twenty-five patients to see then you**'ve got** twenty-five patients to think about. **So,** it's just trying to get, to get the **balance. What I'm saying is,** sometimes you get the **balance** right, hopefully most times you get the **balance** right, sometimes you don't. {You've got to live with that. You've got to live with that.}
> J: {Yeah. Yeah. It's like in any . . . }
> Dr.: **You know,** you've just got to live with it and accept that it might happen and hope, **you know,** the opportunity arrives subsequently [?] to almost remedy the situation.

One can see in this excerpt which discursive strategies this GP employs to "persuade" me of his point of view. First of all, the GP prepares himself physically to put forward his argument by clearing his throat. Throughout the passage the GP uses "you know" a number of times to establish a participatory framework with me. I supported this strategy by using the back channels "yeah, yeah," which indicate to the speaker that his argument is followed by the listener. The GP's style is highly affirmative, as can be seen in the interjection "yes" ("when you think in terms of each individual patient then yes, you're obviously concerned") and in the numerous repetitions of the auxiliary verb "have got to," which emphasize the GP's absolute and unquestionable obligation to consider all his patients equally: "you really have got to think what you do," "When you've got a surgery of twenty-five patients to see then you've got twenty-five patients to think about." The argumentation is also marked by syntactic parallelism ("when you think," "when you've got," and "sometimes you get the balance right, hopefully most times you get the balance right") as well as by the repetition of important lexical items such as "balance." In using all these discourse features the GP creates what Tannen (1989) calls a "high-involvement style," that is, a style that aims at involving both speaker and listener to the greatest possible extent in talk-in-interaction. That this strategy is successful in this example can be seen in the speech overlap:

> {You've got to live with that. You've got to live with that.}
> {Yeah, yeah. It's like in any . . . }

I tried to make a supportive comment and was so keen that I overlapped the interviewee's argumentation by prematurely taking up my next turn. Again, this shows that oral narratives are contextually situated and that their linguistic shape is inevitably influenced by the given situation. In my analyses I comment on similar features of talk-in-interaction where they quite noticeably had an impact on narrative construction.

Let me now turn to the actual data of my study. In the next chapter I commence by presenting interview materials against which the subsequent narratives are shown to deviate in content and structure.

4. Signs of Abuse
"Classic" Disclosures and Narrative Trajectories

Narrative research is sometimes criticized for focusing on certain types of data while neglecting others. Some anthropologists, for example, are concerned that social action may be oversimplified when interpreted in narrative terms and that "a focus on narrative may blind the researcher to the nonverbal aspects of meaning in cultural action" (Mattingly 2000:188). While other qualitative methods such as grounded theory and participant observation, for example, take into account all the data elicited and transcribed for a piece of research, narrative research inevitably leaves out large parts of a sample in order to concentrate on material that is specifically narrative in nature. Some may argue, and perhaps justifiably, that this selective approach can introduce bias into analysis and results. However, as Riessman points out, narratives "are interpretive and, in turn, require interpretation," while "analytic interpretations are partial, alternative truths" (1993:22). I have made every effort to use all the interview material where applicable rather than only the narratives on their own in order to provide a bigger picture of what the GPs had to say about domestic violence. For the same reason I also introduce what one could consider "normalizing" data in this chapter, that is, data from the interviews against the background of which the narratives in my sample can be demonstrated to deviate in intriguing ways. In particular, I look at the signs and symptoms GPs discussed as relevant indicators for domestic violence issues, possible forms of disclosure in consultations, and narrative trajectories concerning both the patient's life story and the story of the (non)disclosure.

Signs and Symptoms
One of the questions I asked during the interviews concerned possible signs or symptoms that would indicate to the doctors that domestic violence might be an issue for a patient. The GPs in my sample answered this question from two per-

spectives: the way domestic violence came out into the open and indicators of the problem that might not necessarily lead to disclosure. Thus, a GP could distinguish between overt and covert forms of presentation. Doctors spoke about patients being "up front" concerning the problem or about "oblique presentations," for example. The signs or symptoms of abuse can in turn be divided into physical or psychological ones. Physical signs like marks and bruises, broken bones, black eyes, and so on are fairly obvious unless hidden under clothes, while psychological symptoms are harder to identify and, if identified, may not necessarily lead to the suspicion and detection of a domestic violence background. It is not inappropriate or even immoral for doctors to go by physical symptoms. However, in the case of psychosocial problems such as domestic violence, to go by physical symptoms alone can be detrimental, as causes of illness may remain opaque, and therefore treatment may be ineffective. If nonphysical symptoms are deliberately overlooked for reasons of fear, helplessness, or lack of interest, then I think doctors' moral stance in domestic violence cases ought to come under closer scrutiny and be challenged. Even though we have to acknowledge that general practitioners are perhaps not in a position to treat the causes or prevent the effects of domestic violence, they are nevertheless gatekeepers to salient help resources and as such have a moral responsibility to leave the gates open. As I discussed in chapter 3, women might disclose domestic violence to their GPs because their periodic, intimate, and physical contact offers occasions for disclosure even without physical symptoms. Recognizing this potential and working toward improvement in the health service provision to battered women is imperative if we seriously wish to tackle the problem.

The GPs' responses yield a number of results with regard to possible signs of abuse. I conducted a type and token analysis on the interview transcripts, drawing up a list of "typical" signs that recurred in the GPs' responses and for which I counted the tokens, that is, the number of occurrences of each type, across the interviews. For each respondent I counted each mentioned type only once, even though some types may have been mentioned several times during the interview or may have contained various subtypes. The types of signs are either physical or psychological. I attached general labels or headings to each subcategory, under which I then subsumed the GPs' various responses. Thus, under physical symptoms I included physical symptoms such as the ones mentioned above (marks, bruises, etc.); unexplained injury, that is, injuries that were not compat-

Physical symptoms	Number of mentions	Psychological symptoms	Number of mentions
Physical symptoms (bruises, black eyes, etc.)	11	Psychiatric/psychological illness	2
Unexplained injury	7	Depression	12
Physical symptoms on children	2	Psychosomatic disturbances	4
		Sleeplessness	3
		Nervousness, anxiety	4
		Emotional problems	7
		Relationship problems	8
		Alcohol or drug abuse	4
		Change of behavior	2
Totals:	20		46

ible with the story the patient provided or that "didn't add up," as one GP put it; and physical injuries on children, which pointed toward a violent background in the home. The psychological symptoms include psychological or psychiatric illness in general; depression; psychosomatic disturbances such as stomach pains; nervousness and anxiety; sleeplessness; relationship problems or, in the words of one of the doctors, "domestic unhappiness"; emotional problems such as distress, being upset, irritability, and stress in general; alcohol or drug abuse in the women as a result of domestic violence; change of behavior; and low self-esteem or confidence. The count yielded the figures shown in table 2.

What is interesting in these findings is that physical symptoms, although they were mentioned by most GPs (eleven GPs mentioned physical symptoms, seven mentioned unexplained injury, and two referred to physical symptoms on children as signs of domestic abuse), are clearly outweighed by the number of psychological symptoms the GPs listed (forty-six mentions of psychological symptoms in comparison with twenty mentions of physical signs). This shows that GPs are aware of the fact that domestic abuse need not present itself overtly but is in fact often hidden among a range of other problems. This could also be seen in the forms of disclosure the GPs discussed. Thus, twelve GPs said that women were fairly up front if they wanted to disclose and simply admit that domestic violence was an issue, while the same number of GPs conjured up scenarios where women came into the practice with something else, with minor problems or even presenting their children rather than themselves. As the GPs contended, this kind of covert presentation usually went on for some time before the actual problem came out or the women felt ready to reveal their real reason for coming. Two doctors maintained that in most cases the problem was disclosed in retrospect, often long after the actual incident, and often at moments when the woman had already decided to leave her partner, for example. Some GPs mentioned as a special form of overt presentation cases where either other members of the health care team such as nurses or health visitors alerted the GPs to possible violence or where family members of patients reported that their mother, daughter, or other female relative suffered abuse from her partner.

Interestingly enough, only five of the thirty-six actual narratives in the sample explicitly mention or provide examples of psychological and/or verbal abuse (narratives 2, 7, 27, 30, 33). This stands in stark contrast to the general responses GPs offered when asked about signs of abuse. It looks as though knowledge about signs and symptoms is theoretical and stored in a more schematized knowledge repertoire, while the instantiations of this knowledge in narratives of practical experiences reveal a much narrower conceptual context, with an emphasis on physical signs. In other words, while GPs know about nonphysical presentations, their practice experience seems to be largely founded on cases where physical violence was an issue and where the resulting physical marks brought that violence to their attention or facilitated the woman's disclosure. As one young male GP commented:

> 1. Well, sometimes you just get an inkling that there's, you know, relationship problems through, er, what the patient actually tells you herself, you know, they usually, invariably they're open in saying, you know, "my husband," or, you know, "he has hit me in the past." And they're, they tend to be more on the timid side when they present like that, um, whereas the ones [laughs] who come in with black eyes and things tend to be the aggressive type.

Put differently, women who present physical injuries are more likely to disclose violence, as the signs are obvious to the GP, whereas in cases with nonphysical signs the abuse may go unnoticed unless the woman opens up. The following response by a young female GP is telling in this respect:

> 2. Um, occasionally you come across funny bruises and things, very occasionally that would happen. Um, it's more likely to be somebody who's coming in feeling stressed and depressed and when you

ask more about it, um, they may hint and then you can enquire further, but some of them will come in and tell you, you know, it's their
husband or whatever, but not many.

This GP clearly identifies psychological or emotional problems as triggers for
suspicion, but again, unless the woman is prepared to volunteer further information ("they **may** hint"), domestic violence may not be established as the
cause of these problems.

Even when there are physical signs, women may not be willing to open up.
One late-middle-aged male GP, when asked about indicators, responded:

3. Well, the type of injury, obviously, and the circumstances the patient comes in, that they'd been nervous, not willing to, er, go to
casualty, er, not willing to discuss how the injury came about or
they give you some daft story, or there's more than one person in
the household who's got bruises, like the child, if there was a child,
that's what I think, there's lots of, just if there was a change of behavior in the patient as well to a certain extent, um, er, you know,
these things are all, they're just indicators. **There's nothing, unless
somebody says that they'd been assaulted you can't be a hundred
percent certain of anything, can you?**

Does this uncertainty warrant GPs' lack of action or reluctance to probe the issue further? The following response by a middle-aged female GP suggests that
doctors might indeed act along the lines of such reasoning:

4. I mean, yeah, I mean I'm, yeah, I think, um, if it's someone you're
seeing a lot and, you know, you're, you feel you're just on the brink
of something, **there's times where obviously you think this is going to just cause ripples.** And, and, yeah, I mean I think you're always [?] you've got to feel that they're ready to deal with it as well
'cause, er, you know, **if you challenge patients about it they may not
be ready to face what you're, what you're saying** 'cause of the way
they've been living so, I think, if, if they come up with it, it's different. **If you've got a hunch then you're probably waiting to pick up
the right cues about when is the right time.** If you don't think it is, I
think you would, you know, in a way we collude with them slightly, I

think, until they're ready to talk about it because it may make things worse if you challenge someone that, you know, "I think this is happening at home. Do you want to tell me about it?" **They may never come back if, you know, if you challenge them at the wrong time** and I think it's, it's, it's, difficult 'cause you might be wrong even when you decide to talk about it but I think you've got to maybe try and pick up when they're ready. And, to be honest, it seems to be more when there's a crisis and then they come to you and then you can say, "Well, you know, I'm really glad you, you said that. **I've had a suspicion but I wanted to wait for, for you to tell me,**" so, you know, that, that's, that tends to be the pattern. Mmm.

This response already raises a number of issues that I address in more detail in the subsequent chapters, issues concerning agency, responsibility, moral implications, anxiety, doctor-patient relationship, sensitivity, time, role definitions, and so on. The response thus also shows that disclosure of domestic violence in general practice is a highly complex topic and that in order to even begin to understand its complexity we have to pay closer attention to the interplay of the issues involved. It is not least for this reason that a narrative investigation into the discursive encoding and construction of domestic violence in general practice is a suitable method, as it allows a GP to attend to particularities in life experiences and, more important, to the affective side of such particularities. This can be seen, for example, in the last GP's reenactment of part of a (fictive) consultation by means of direct discourse, which is a feature that recurs frequently throughout the interviews and in the narratives in particular. By using direct discourse the GP brings the doctor-patient encounter to life within the interview and thus emphasizes her own emotional state, which she imparted to her patient in the consultation and later indirectly to me, the interviewer: "I'm really glad you said that."

"Standard" Scenarios

The response in (4) is also interesting as it relates a scene of disclosure that this GP considered common or, as she said, that "tends to be the pattern." Other GPs made similar statements about "standard" presentations. Consider the following responses:

5. a. Some will come up very up front [fortunately ?], saying that they've been beaten up. Some will do the **classic introduction that they come with something very minor**

b. [Sighs] I suppose **one of the classical indications from a** GP's **point of view is, er, a pattern of unexplained and recurring, er, injury.** Um, possibly a, either in addition or separately, a history of, er, emotional, oblique psychiatric illness, um, or unexplained psychosomatic, er, conditions. Er, relationship problems in the home, particularly with the children, er, someone becoming more introspective, er, these are some things that might alert me. [Only] still the best one, I think, is possibly a pattern of [?] unexplained or badly explained, er, injuries.

c. Um, [pause] I'm trying to just think back, um, the things I've seen, er, very often it's, rather than being an acute situation and someone's been, been attacked, er, **it may come out in, you know, later, later discussions of, where they're presenting with some sort of emotional distress, um, I think that's, that's a normal, the normal sort of way we come, get to know about it.** Occasionally people come in and present their, their bruises but, er, yeah. Um, there's, [there are], usually it's wives involved, there, I think there's the odd occasion of a, er, er, some older people being, being, well, claiming they've been attack—— or alleging they've been attacked by relatives. That sometimes happens so, but, er, as I say, but it, la——, **largely it's just in, in retrospect rather than at an acute stage.**

d. Okay. It's usually, I would say, **usually one of two ways, er, it, it can present. It may be that the woman turns up at the surgery with an appointment, er, either on an urgent basis or as part of a routine appointment, and will usually in the course of the consultation say that she wants to, um, confide that she's been abused.** Um, often it isn't the first time that they discuss it, they will often come in maybe later on in the consultation, um, and in that situation, obviously, um, we listen, we record what happened, we record any injuries, I um, and **the other way that, er, that they present is in retrospect** through the solicitors, when we get a letter in from the solicitor saying that this lady perhaps wants a divorce or is gonna be separated from her husband on the basis that he's been violent towards her and can we provide any record of that and, sometimes we have a record of that incident and [if] we don't, um, so, ach, that's probably one of the commonest way it presents.

e. I mean the other thing which is fairly straightforward is if you have evidence of physical violence and they come for that and they say: **"Oh, I ran against the door." Typical thing to say when they have got a black eye** and I've never seen, you don't get a black eye from running against the doors, it's just mechanically not really possible.
J: Yeah?
Dr.: Yeah. Um, then, but then it would be obvious very often, I don't think that, that patients very often present with that. Then it's, but then it's [virtually] straightforward although I could imagine that then there might be a temptation for GPs to overlook that and take the evidence at face value and, and send them away because it's more convenient than touching on the, the underlying thing.

f. Um, but **mostly it's, it's the, the scenario that things aren't, that the patients have said things aren't going well and they'll tell you that the, their partner sometimes hits them,** say, when they're drunk or, or that sort of thing. Sometimes they'll tell you in retrospect, you know, that they've left him because obviously he was just **"lifting the hand," that's always what they say up here.** "He was lifting his hand and, um, that's why I left." And, um, that's quite common as well that they sometimes don't want to tell you actually at the time. Sometimes they do.

Given these responses, "common" presentations of domestic violence cases seem to include one or more of the following features: covert presentations, whereby the women come to the practice allegedly for some other reason, as in (5a) and (5d); physical symptoms that remain unexplained or for which the women make up a false story, as in (5b) and (5e); violence disclosed in retrospect rather than at an acute stage, as in (5c), (5d), and (5f); overt presentation, where the woman voluntarily broaches the topic, as in (5f). I must add the caveat that it is very difficult to gauge what exactly a "standard" presentation of domestic violence in general practice is, as the concept will always be based on what GPs and patients tell an interviewer rather than on observed doctor-patient consultations. Thus, "standard" presentations are themselves discursively constructed concepts, just as domestic violence itself is to a certain extent discursively and culturally constructed. In the above examples this can be seen in the use of euphemisms such as "lifting the hand" (5f) and in redefinitions of violence such as "ran against the door" (5e).

What is intriguing with regard to more global narrative structures, however, is the fact that only a few of the GPs' narratives of real practice encounters with domestic violence victims follow the pattern of the "standard" scenario the GPs discussed elsewhere in the interview. As the analyses in subsequent chapters demonstrate, many of the narratives, albeit not all of them, depict cases where the violence was not presented in retrospect but at an acute stage when the physical symptoms played a major part in detection and treatment. In fact, a number of GPs related incidents they had come across while working in emergency rooms rather than in general practice. Other narratives depict surprising and unexpected disclosures after lengthy periods during which the GPs were unaware of the possibility of domestic violence. This combines covert presentation with disclosure in retrospect, albeit with a rather passive part played by the GP. Yet other narratives do not deal so much with the disclosure itself as with the pangs of frustration and helplessness GPs experienced once a domestic violence case had come out into the open and they felt inadequately equipped to deal with it. In other words, what is also missing in much of my data is "hero stories," that is, narratives about successful encounters between doctors and battered women.

One of the problems underlying this finding, I contend, is a general mismatch of narrative trajectories. Young observes that "physicians characteristically treat storytelling as an interruption of, distraction from, or incursion into the realm of medicine" (1997:68). In cases of domestic violence the narrative trajectory of the woman's life story often does not overlap with or sufficiently feed into the trajectory of the medical consultation, that is, the story of the encounter between doctor and patient within the practice environment. This undoubtedly also has to do with cultural expectations of what can be told in certain situations. Frank points out for illness narratives in general: "From their families and friends, from the popular culture that surrounds them, and from the stories of other ill people, storytellers have learned formal structures of narrative, conventional metaphors and imagery, and standards of what is and is not appropriate to tell" (1995:3). Thus, women may feel that it is not appropriate to tell their GP about their abusive relationship, especially if the GP does not give the impression that he or she is receptive to such a narrative.

Narrative Trajectories

The term "narrative trajectories" is widely used in the study of life narratives and biographies. Some of the most prominent representatives in the field are Anselm Strauss and Barney Glaser. I mainly draw upon the work of the German sociologist Fritz Schütze (1981, 1983), whose research is informed by Strauss's and Glaser's work. Schütze defines social trajectories as very dense, conditional (but not intentional) chains of events that display a global sequential structure (1981:90–91). The sequential order of events implies changes in features and definitions of situations of the social unit under investigation, whereby its self-definitions play an important role. This social unit could be an individual person, a group of people, or an organization. Negative trajectories restrict our possibilities for action and development, while positive trajectories open vistas for action and development on the grounds of enhanced possibilities for new social positionings. Action in these concepts is tied to heteronymous conditions, which either increase and thereby cause the social subject to lose control or decrease and thus augment our power of action. At certain points in life trajectories we can identify action schemas (i.e., ways people deal with given situations), which have an impact on the progress and direction of these trajectories. Thus, we can talk about initiation, reversal, control, interpretation, normalization, and end. These action schemas can be in the hands of the social individual or people in this individual person's social surroundings, for example, friends, family, and colleagues.

Illness narratives can also be analyzed with regard to their trajectories and their impact on wider life trajectories. Frank (1995), for example, describes patterns of illness narratives in terms of a range of plot lines: the "quest narrative," the "restitution narrative," the "chaos narrative," for example. A problem arises in doctor-patient interaction, Schütze argues, when the professional, that is, the doctor, does not leave room for the patient's hesitation in decision taking (e.g., with regard to treatment options) and thus infringes on the patient's autonomy for action:

> Geht der Professionelle—gerade aus technologisch orientierten Rationalisierungsvorstellungen heraus—nicht in dieser Weise auf die Entscheidungsautonomie des Klienten ein, wird die handlungsschematische Aktivitätsstruktur des Klienten als betroffenen Biographieträger vollends gebrochen. Er wird dann zu einem passiven Objekt professionellen Handelns degradiert, das in den Handlungsvorgaben des Professionellen nur noch gehorchen, reagieren und erleiden kann, dessen Eigenaktivitäten also überhaupt nicht mehr adäquat unter dem Leitgesichtspunkt intentionalen Handelns analysieren [sic] werden können. (Schütze 1981:87)
>
> [If the professional, for reasons of technologically oriented concepts of rationalization, does not thus take notice of the client's autonomy in decision taking, the structure of the client's action schemas as the person telling his or her biography is disrupted. He or she is then downgraded to a passive object of professional action who can only listen to, react, and suffer within the action rules set up by the professional and whose own activities can therefore no longer be adequately analyzed under the main aspect of intentional action. (my translation)]

In other words, if patients' biographies and life stories are pressed into a temporally and narratively restricted professional framework such as the consultation, the patient's autonomy regarding the telling and shaping of his or her life story at this point is also limited. The same applies to consultations in which domestic violence is an issue. Battered women bring to the consultation a whole gamut of experiences, their personal life trajectories, which may not fit into the somewhat limited trajectory of the medical encounter. In order to illustrate this point I discuss the problem of narrative trajectories in greater detail in one of the narratives of my sample.

The "Cloak-and-Dagger Stuff"

Six of the thirty-six narratives in my sample tell stories of women who managed to leave their violent partners. Thus, in narrative 32 the woman eventually

"got rid of her boyfriend"; in narrative 6 it was the danger for the child that finally made the woman leave her violent partner; in narrative 25 an older woman
moved away from home after many years of violence; narrative 36 relates the
story of a patient who had already contacted a lawyer because she was planning
to sue her husband (although the outcome of this is never established in the
narrative); and narratives 10 and 12 relate stories in which the women went to
hostels. Let us take a closer look at one of these "success stories":

Narrative 10

1. =Oh, I do remember.
2. I do remember.
3. An amazing case.
4. Yes, I had an amazing case in casualty once when, um,
   somebody had, um,
5. that was a long time ago,
6. somebody had come in
7. and obviously had been, you know, really quite badly beaten
   up
8. and was terrified to, to go home.
9. And her partner arrived in casualty at the front door,
   demanding to see her.
10. Um, and we didn't know what to do really
11. and what we did,
12. we phoned Women's Aid
13. and we spoke to this amazing lady who has now retired.
14. She was a, a professor's wife at the hospital, um,
15. and she arranged everything.
16. And she, it was almost as the cloak-and-dagger stuff,
17. she appeared in the back door and smuggled this woman out.
18. Then she went to the hostel.

The narrative relates a consultation in an emergency room. Even before she starts
her narrative the GP evaluates it by calling the case "amazing," which she reinforces later in the narrative by likening what happened to the "cloak-and-dagger stuff." This is interesting, as it suggests that, first, helping a woman escape
her violent partner is not something doctors normally do and, second, the res-

cue was experienced by the GP as something almost "unreal," or like an adventure story found on TV or in popular fiction. The overall structure of the narrative coincides with what we could classify as the commonly expected narrative trajectory in medical encounters: presentation, treatment, cure. Thus, the orientation sequence in lines 1 to 8 not only provides background information on time ("a long time ago"), place ("in casualty"), and characters ("I" and "somebody") but, medically speaking, presents a case, typically through physical symptoms: the woman was "really quite badly beaten up" (line 7). In the complicating action sequence in lines 9 to 14 the medical staff, faced with the violent partner's threatening intrusion, take action to help the woman: "we phoned Women's Aid and we spoke to this amazing lady" (lines 12 and 13). This parallels the process of "treatment" in medical encounters. The result of this "treatment" is "cure": thus, in the narrative's resolution, the doctors manage to "smuggle" the woman out of the hospital and help her move into a hostel and leave her violent partner. Admittedly, the comparison is flawed, as it is not, strictly speaking, "medical" intervention that helps the woman in the end. Furthermore, we do not learn whether the woman stayed in the hostel or what happened to her after that. This is exactly where the problem for medical narratives surfaces: the lack or insufficiency of the woman's life story for the doctor.

In narrative 10 we learn nothing about the woman's previous life and the circumstances of her violent relationship. What was her socioeconomic situation? Did she have friends and family? What was her relationship like? Were they married? How did her partner abuse her? Likewise, there is no information on what happened after the woman went to the hostel. Did she find herself a place of her own? Did her partner leave her alone or threaten her? Did she divorce him (if they were married)? Did she go back to him? It is this lack of additional information about the women's life stories that makes the GPs' narratives an unsatisfactory genre. Put differently, the lamination of the narrative trajectories of the women's stories and the medical narrative trajectories is mostly incomplete. This incompleteness, I argue, underlies much of the problems general practitioners encounter in consultations where domestic violence is an issue.

We might object here that the lack of additional information about the woman can be attributed more to the fact that this narrative was told in an interview rather than to problems underlying doctor-patient conversation. However, Trinch (2003) demonstrates how battered women's stories are transformed in institutional settings—in her study, legal institutions—in order to fit the fairly rigid genres of affidavit and protective order application. Trinch contends that "this imposition of one genre on the other causes fragmentation in women's stories that leaves them open-ended and even vulnerable to discrepancy" (2003:215). As the analyses of the narratives in this book show, it is precisely the discrepancy between divergent teleological directions of the women's and the doctors' stories in addition to inherent differences in the framing and fashioning of the narratives themselves that lead to difficulties in doctor-patient relationships concerning the disclosure of domestic violence, as I mentioned in chapter 3. In the following chapters I demonstrate to what extent GPs' telling of their stories within a biomedical framework, their discursive constructions of space and time, of agency and role definitions may impede successful outcomes of consultations with women suffering domestic abuse.

Before I move on to more detailed analyses, however, let me introduce briefly another narrative from my sample that stands out in terms of its overall structure and with regard to its component narrative trajectories.

Narrative 30

1. She, well, she's interesting.
2. She's a schiz——, she's labeled as a schizophrenic
3. but she's not, she's not really, she's not, er, particularly bad in that way
4. and she lives, um, in a flat she has bought
5. and she has a partner who she wants to get out of the flat, who's really ins——, er, installed himself in there and [has lived] there for a number of years
6. and, um, he, er, er, he's, er, mentally and physically abusive towards her
7. and, um, he really just, er, pushes her around
8. and makes her do all the shopping,
9. he makes her carry everything,
10. he turns off all the lights and the telly when he wants it off,
11. he changes the TV program if he doesn't like it on,
12. and he resorts to physical violence
13. **and, and she came in the other week, last week, with a big black eye and some bruising**

14. and then I had a chat with her about it
15. and, er, [she felt ashamed]
16. and then, before I suspected it
17. I'd never actually known that he's been physically abusive
18. but, er, she obviously is unhappy with him
19. but can't get him out of the flat.
20. He pays rent
21. and he's fairly, er, aggressive [?].
22. She likes to watch some television program,
23. he prefers if she puts it, the, the nasty, aggressive things on the telly.
24. So she's in a bit of a dilemma
25. and, being mentally unwell, she, she hasn't worked for a number of years,
26. she doesn't have, um, she, she's not very skilled at times to or-gani——, to manage this situation.
27. She does have support from the CPN [clinical psychiatric nurse]
28. but I don't think, er,
29. it's very difficult to know how best to help her actually 'cause
30. I said to her last week she should go to, to seek legal advice.
31. I suggested that she maybe goes to the Citizens Advice first to get some help with that.
32. She's not, well, financially, she's badly off
33. so she's worried about all sorts of legal fees.
34. I suggested to her that one option might be to come out of the flat and seek refuge
35. and then [the Citizens Advice section] will get him out
36. but she understandably is reluctant to do that because it's her flat,
37. she actually pays the mortgage
38. and he pays her rent.
39. That's pretty minimal
40. but he does.
41. So she's in a very unhappy situation

42. and she really doesn't want to get involved with him
43. but she can't get rid of him.
    J: All right. But she was fairly up front about the {problem?}
Dr.:   {Very, yeah.}
44. Well, I've known her for quite a, about ten years or so, she
45. and, er, with her schizophrenic illness it's taken awhile getting her to talk about things
46. but she's actually quite well from that point of view,
47. she's not psychotic at all at the moment
48. and I don't think, er, that's an issue.
49. I think there's an issue in that she is not very good at managing the situation and,
50. and she's, and she's not working,
51. she's only forty-six
52. but she's not working.
53. She has no other financial, er, input of actual benefits.
54. **Um, but I mean it was obvious when she had the black eye that, that she'd been assaulted**
55. **but she was quite moved from that how it happened**
56. **and she did say this wasn't a new thing,**
57. **it happened several times in the past.**

Narrative 30 obviously does not represent a typical Labovian oral narrative. First of all, it employs both present and past tense rather than only the more common past tense, and it also deviates from the diamond pattern in that its overall structure is cyclical and repetitive, which makes the narrative much longer. I have marked the parts that can be considered the "narrative proper" about the consultation in bold type to illustrate its fragmentary and repetitive nature. The protagonist of the story had already been briefly mentioned earlier in the interview, which accounts for the fact that the GP starts his narrative with the anaphoric personal pronoun "she." The lengthy orientation section in lines 2 to 6 provides background information on the patient's schizophrenic illness, her relationship, and her violent partner. Interestingly enough, this background information is supplemented and thus made more vivid by a list of examples of domestic violence as perpetrated by the patient's partner: "he really just, er, pushes her around and makes her do all the shopping, he makes her carry everything, he turns off all the lights and the telly when he wants it off, he changes the TV program if he doesn't like it on, and he resorts to physical violence" (lines 7 to 12). What strikes us as unusual here compared to all the other narratives in the sample is the amount of detail with which the GP depicts domestic violence. Physical violence appears as only one form of abuse among a whole range of mainly emotional types of violence, which indicates that the doctor acknowledges not only the physical or "medical" side of the patient's problem but also the emotional and mental implications, as can be seen in the GP's own classification of the partner's violence: "he's, er, *mentally* and physically abusive towards her" (line 6, my emphasis).

Information about the patient's background is repeatedly and extensively brought up in the narrative (lines 18–21, 24–27, 32–33, 36–43, and 44–53), and it centers around the following major themes: the patient's schizophrenia, her resulting lack of ability "to manage the situation" (line 26), which ties in with the woman's unemployment and thus her financial dependence on her violent partner. Although other doctors in the sample also mentioned women's deviant behavior as part of domestic violence, whether as a reason or a consequence, this doctor is very cautious when talking about his patient's illness. The self-repair in line 2 indicates a high degree of self-consciousness in the interview as well as an awareness of the problem of labeling: "She's a schiz——, she's labeled as a schizophrenic." Instead of immediately attaching the label "schizophrenic" to his patient, the doctor metalinguistically refers to labels, and he explicitly emphasizes several times during the narrative that the illness is not an issue for the patient and, more important, that it does not relate causally to the violence the woman suffers: "she's not, er, particularly bad in that way" (line 3); "but she's actually quite well from that point of view, she's not psychotic at all at the moment and I don't think, er, that's an issue" (lines 46–48).

Where the GP draws a causal connection, however, is between the woman's illness and the fact that she does not work, which, in turn, contributes to her financial dependence on her partner and her inability to cope with the situation. The causal relationship is linguistically conveyed through the close collocation of clauses expressing these aspects: "being mentally unwell, she, she hasn't worked for a number of years, she doesn't have, um, she, she's not very skilled at times to organi——, to manage this situation" (lines 25–26); "I think there's an issue in that she is not very good at managing the situation and, and she's, and she's not working, she's only forty-six but she's not working. She has no other financial, er, input of actual benefits" (lines 49–53). The financial situation is mentioned as a crucial factor that hinders the woman from leaving her violent partner or getting him out of her flat. Again, the clauses used to describe the situation are strikingly similar and repetitive: "she has a partner who she wants to get out of the flat, who's really ins——, er, installed himself in there" (line 5); "she obviously is unhappy with him but can't get him out of the flat. He pays rent" (lines 18–20); "she understandably is reluctant to do that [i.e., leave the flat] because it's her flat, she actually pays the mortgage and he pays her rent. That's pretty minimal but he does" (lines 36–40); "she can't get rid of him" (line 43). What emerges is a fairly complex picture of a relationship in which both external and internal pressures keep the woman from leaving her partner.

Detail and Narrative Trajectories

The fact that this GP has such detailed knowledge of all the circumstances so that he is able to relate them in an elaborate narrative indicates two things: first, the woman's own narrative must have been very elaborate, which shows that there must have been sufficient time for narrative production in the consultation; second, the GP displays great interest in his patient's case and the underlying circumstances because he considers them "reportable" enough to present them in the interview to such an extent. The woman's narrative trajectory was projected into the consultation and was then to some extent mapped onto the interview I conducted with the GP. The GP even displayed awareness of the patient's feelings during the consultation: "she felt ashamed" (line 15); "she was quite moved from that" (line 55). The actual narrative about the consultation during which the patient finally opened up about her problem is thus enriched by an array of circumstantial information that is missing from most of the other narratives. Interestingly enough, however, the narrative proper here, which also stands out through the use of past tense, shares more common features with the other narratives. The core of the story is the GP's surprise when he hears for the first time that domestic violence occurs in the woman's relationship: "and then, before I suspected it, I'd never actually known that he's been physically abusive" (lines 16–17). It is astonishing that this comes out after the woman has lived with her partner "for a number of years" (line 5), and, as in some of the other narratives, the trigger for disclosure is a physical sign of abuse: "and she came in the other week, last week, with a big black eye and some bruising" (line 13). Physical signs thus again appear to be more easily identifiable in general practice and are more likely to raise suspicion in the GP. They form part of the typical "story skeleton" (Schank 1990) of most of the GPs' narratives in my sample. Nevertheless, narrative 30 differs from most of the other stories in that it allows for the unfolding of the trajectory of the woman's life story within the medical narrative trajectory.

We can speculate now to what extent this may further sensitize the GP or make him more alert in future consultations. I venture to argue here that the more scope is given to women's life narrative trajectories within consultations, the more likely disclosure of domestic violence is to take place. As far as doctors' narrative knowledge about domestic violence is concerned, this also implies that the more complex GPs' story skeletons about domestic violence cases are, the more knowledge these GPs will be able to retrieve in another consultation where this knowledge may become relevant. However, as I said earlier, most of the narratives in my sample present a different picture. It is to these narratives that I now turn in greater detail.

5. Setting the Scene of Abuse

Metaphors and Spatiotemporal Mapping

In this chapter I investigate how GPs linguistically create spatiotemporal and other metaphorical frameworks for their narratives and to what extent these frameworks indicate mental images that reveal the GPs' perceptions and definitions of domestic violence, on the one hand, and of their own work in general practice, on the other. I present how GPs verbalize their encounters with domestic violence victims in the consultation room and in what ways time and space influence their relationships with patients.

Metaphorical language has been a central point of discussion ever since Aristotle's poetics, and opinions on the purpose and functioning of metaphors have been diverse. Scholars from a variety of disciplines such as literary studies (Birus 2000; Wellbery 1997), linguistics (Ortony 1993), cognitive science, anthropology (Celi and Boiero 2002), and language philosophy (Stern 2000) continue to contribute varied and fascinating insights into both the use and meaning of metaphor. I adopt Turner's definition of metaphor: "Metaphor consists of the employment of an attribute of a given semantic domain as a predication or representation of an attribute of a different domain, on the basis of a perceived similarity between the two attributes" (1991:121). The concept that is expressed in different terms is often called the "tenor" or "topic"; the term that expresses it is called the "vehicle." The perceived similarity or common quality underlying both expressions is sometimes referred to as *tertium comparationis*, that is, the "third [element] of the comparison."

Like narrative, metaphor can be considered from a realist perspective as originating from a process of "resonating to perceptual information in the world" (Dent-Read and Szokolszky 1993:227), or it can be defined in constructionist terms as "a sui generis mode of giving form and identity to the otherwise inchoate experience (at least, experience of self-identity) of phenomenological subjects" (Turner 1991:126). In other words, metaphors are rooted in the "real world" to the extent that tenor and vehicle are usually derived from existing and well-known things or concepts. On the other hand, metaphors construct new and often multiple meanings and thereby invite interpretation. Stern points out that "it is our semantic knowledge of the character of a metaphor that enables us to express knowledge and information by the metaphor in addition to that expressed in its (propositional) content (in context)" (2000:261). Metaphors may thus convey attitudes toward and feelings about a given issue. As Kirmayer maintains, "each type of trope achieves its effect by presenting the listener with information that can be used to construct some set of implications that are relevant to the speaker's implied intentions" (2000:177). If one follows this line of reasoning, it should become clear why an investigation into the use of metaphors in GPs' discourse on domestic violence is essential: not only do the metaphors doctors use to describe victims and perpetrators tell us something about their (unconscious) attitudes toward and feelings about these people, but the same metaphors may give us an indication of how these doctors perceive their own embodiment in their professional domain, which may in turn point toward ways in which they interact with their patients on a day-to-day basis. After all, metaphors may well become "self-fulfilling prophecies" (Lakoff and Johnson 1980:156) in the sense that people accommodate to the "truth" and the coherent experience they perceive in these metaphors.

Some scholars have focused on the cognitive dimension of metaphor. Thus, Lakoff and Johnson (1980) maintain that human thought processes are largely metaphorical, and Lakoff's (1993) concept of "cross-domain mapping" captures the process by which people comprehend one mental domain in terms of another. Lakoff defines the term "metaphorical expression" as "a linguistic expression (a word, phrase, or sentence) that is the surface realization of such a cross-domain mapping" (1993:203). Metaphors therefore determine to a large extent our understanding of the world, as Lakoff and Johnson maintain: "What is real for an individual as a member of a culture is a product both of his social reality and of the way in which that shapes his experience of the physical world. Since much of our social reality is understood in metaphorical terms, and since our conception of the physical world is partly metaphorical, metaphor plays a very significant role in determining what is real for us" (1980:146).

The assumption is that metaphoricity is out of awareness and therefore indicative of unconscious dispositions, which in Lakoff and Johnson's model of em-
bodied reality consist of body sets. In other words, the roots of metaphor can
be found in the body and one's experiences of physical processes. Thus, for example, it is very common for people to say "I feel *low*" or "*down*" when their
overall emotional state is negative because this state is associated with a slop-
ing physical posture, while to feel good can be expressed in statements such as
"I'm on a *high* today," a feeling that goes along with an upright body position.
What is at stake here is that originally spatial terms have come to be used for
the expression of emotional states.

This cognitive view of metaphor is useful and makes sense on introspec-
tion of our own use of language, yet we must not forget that metaphors are also
culturally and socially situated and are ultimately expressions of culture. Even
seemingly "obvious" concepts such as time and space are in effect culturally
constructed. The ethnographic works by Sapir and Whorf provide early examples of the ways different cultures conceptualize and, consequently, verbalize time and space differently. Metaphors furthermore need to be considered
more locally within the discourse context out of which they emerge. As Cameron points out, "processing metaphorical language takes place in context and
draws on the discourse expectations of participants" (1999:25). Since "it is precisely the interaction between the cognitive and social in language use that produces the language and behaviour that we observe and research" (Cameron
1999:4), I take the interview and cultural contexts into account where possible in my analyses.

Metaphors are also frequently found in narrative language, since they offer
ways of expressing something differently and less directly. As Prickett points
out in his study on religious and scientific "narratives" produced over the last
three centuries, "the magic of language allows us to formulate metaphors for
aspects of reality that cannot, and never will be, either perceived or directly
approached. . . . Descriptions of something we have not seen rest on analogies
with things we have seen: the first atom bomb was 'brighter than a thousand
suns.' . . . Every metaphor we use . . . is founded on just such a process. They
are all of them, in effect, little narratives" (2002:226–27). Metaphors thus present narrative possibilities. Kirmayer contends that we can articulate ourselves
through metaphor "without appeal to elaborate stories of origins, motives, ob-

stacles, and change," and metaphors thus "may function as gestures toward a story that is not taken up and completed or as reminders of a story that is already authoritative" (2000:155). As I demonstrate below, the reduction of potential narratives to metaphorical expressions can also become problematic in the GPs' discourse on domestic violence.

Spatiotemporal Metaphors

Since spatial imagery forms the foundation of much of metaphorical language in English, I dedicate a considerable part of this chapter to the analysis of such imagery. When people experience the world they are inevitably confronted with the dimensions of time and space. Without a knowledge of space, for example, we would not be able to fulfill seemingly simple tasks such as doing the shopping or getting to our workplace or, more generally, finding our way around places. Downs and Stea refer to people's organized representations of some part of the spatial environment as "cognitive maps" (1977:6), that is, mental images of the environment that have been transformed into, for example, sketch maps showing the route to our house, travel brochures, a list of places we consider dangerous, and children's drawings of their houses and neighborhoods. "Cognitive mapping," by contrast, is the dynamic thought process by which such mental images and models are conjured up, and it is vitally important in the sense that it enables people to know where to go and how to get there. However, cognitive mapping encompasses more than simply a means of orientation. Downs and Stea point out that "in some very fundamental but inexpressible way, our own self-identity is inextricably bound up with knowledge of the spatial environment. We can organize personal experience along the twin dimensions of space and time" (1977:27). In other words, notions of time and space are necessary in our lives because they help us structure mentally not only the environment in which we live but also our everyday experiences of events, encounters with other people, and so on.

If space and time pervade our lives to such an extent as to be vital for our survival, we can assume that space-time parameters are also essential in personal narratives, which are often related to capture and order our life experiences. Herman argues that "such cognitive mapping is fundamental and obligatory for narrative understanding, not a derivative or optional aspect of telling and comprehending stories" (2001:518). Narratives are set within and, at the same time, create a certain "spacetime region" (Herman 2001), that is, the incidents related in narratives are located spatially and temporally, and this spatiotemporal grid is linguistically conveyed to the listener. In the GPS' narratives mainly two locations can be identified: first, the practice environment where the consultation takes place; second, the setting or scene of a violent incident in particular or of violence in general.

Time, the second component of spatiotemporal maps, has received considerable attention from scholars in the social sciences and in narrative research. Labov regards time as one of the most important structural features of oral narratives. He maintains that narratives directly reflect the order of the experienced events in their sequential ordering of clauses: "Narrative, then, is only one way of recapitulating this past experience: the clauses are characteristically ordered in temporal sequence; if narrative clauses are reversed, the inferred temporal sequence of the original semantic interpretation is altered" (Labov 1972a:360). Since, as Herman contends, the study of narrative is "also an inquiry into how modes of storytelling—in particular, strategies for ordering—help shape people's intuitions about what is and what is not the case" (2002:235), the investigation into the time frames of the GPS' narratives presents itself as another important research question.

The GPS' narratives, while themselves located in the given time frame of the interview, also functioned as windows to wider timescapes that constituted the background to their stories of abuse. This is a common feature in oral narratives, as Laurier points out: "Narrative in talk although not detachable from its present situation is part of a shifting out of a narrow and strongly contingent present tense of a conversation to a wider time span that may embed other stories directly or may borrow their formal structurings" (1999:192). Like spatial maps, time can also be considered a metaphor. Adam comments on the use of "time" in our everyday practice and in social science research by emphasizing the difference between clock time and lived, real time: "This socially created, artefactual resource has become so all-embracing that it is now related to as if it were time *per se*, as if there were no other times. . . . The metaphor, in other words, is transposed on to the subject of inquiry and we tend to forget that qualitative variation precedes the uniform, abstract quantity of human origin" (1995:91). In the next chapter I investigate to what extent time can even be mythologized in general practice.

I am aware of the fact that metaphoric expression appears in diverse forms, for example, not only in noun metaphors, which are most commonly used as examples, but also as verbs, prepositions, and so on. The selection of metaphors from a set of discourse data can be difficult, as one has to determine what counts as metaphor and what does not. Many idiomatic expressions (e.g., "We can't turn back now") may not be perceived as metaphors by speakers and have sometimes been classified as "dead metaphors" in the literature, that is, metaphors that are so widely used that they no longer seem to be conspicuous. However, even such idiomatic expressions "do not exist individually as random clichés, but reflect different aspects of our ordinary metaphorical conception" (Gibbs 1999:34) of things. I have mainly applied two criteria to select metaphors: domain incongruity and frequency. Thus, when doctors used expressions from other nonmedical domains to map onto the consultation, for example, these expressions constituted potential candidates for metaphorical analysis. In addition, a number of such expressions recurred frequently throughout the interviews and in various doctors' narratives. To give the reader a flavor of how spatiotemporal mapping bears on the doctors' narratives I start by analyzing one narrative in detail before providing examples of metaphor from the entire sample.

Limitations of the "Medical Gaze"

GPs, although they are probably more familiar with their patients than other doctors, have only a very restricted view of their patients in the confined space-time region of the consultation room. Within a five-to-ten-minute appointment they usually catch mere glimpses of what might be going on in the patient's background. The following narrative related by a middle-aged female GP in a student health center illustrates this restricted field of vision of what Young calls the "deciphering gaze" (1997:83) of doctors in medical examinations. This literal gaze focuses on the deciphering of physical symptoms and is thus embedded in Foucault's (1973) more abstract notion of the "medical gaze," that is, medicine's objectifying visualization and reconceptualization of the body and of patients. The story was told in response to the question "What did you feel at that time?" which referred to a story the GP had told immediately prior to narrative 11. The GP stated that "the problem was that we never knew what happened. You know, you never know how, how things turned out in the long term." Narrative 11 can be regarded as an explanation of this statement.

Narrative 11

1. Um, we had another case here actually.
2. That's, that, we had a little girl who was a drug addict
3. and her boyfriend was a drug addict
4. and that was really sad
5. and she was coming in with black eyes and, you know, bruises and all sorts of things
6. and she was different in that she just couldn't do anything about it.
7. You know, no matter what we suggested
8. she . . . wasn't able to, to break away from this guy.
9. Unless while he was in prison, which was all right, she was much better then
10. and she just, she didn't finish her degree
11. and she just looked iller and iller and more and more tired
12. and eventually she just disappeared
13. and we don't know what's happened to her.
14. She left Aberdeen
15. and goodness knows where she is now.

The narrative begins with an orientation section that comprises lines 1 to 3. By using the indefinite determiner "another" the narrator links the case back to the case she related previously.[1] The GP thus obviously takes advantage of the fact that she has sole power over the floor at this point and uses the opportunity to tell another explanatory story. The narrative proceeds by introducing the protagonists, a girl and her boyfriend, who are both drug addicts. This fact is emphasized through the use of syntactic parallelism in lines 2 and 3, the only difference being that the girl's drug addiction is mentioned in a defining relative clause, while in line 3 the boyfriend's drug addiction forms part of the predicate: "we had a little girl who was a drug addict and her boyfriend was a drug addict." The girl is defined not only in terms of her addiction but also with regard to her physical appearance: she is presented as "little," which automatically evokes a mental image of the girl as being weak or feeble. This image of feebleness is reinforced in lines 6 to 8 and, at the same time, is associated with a lack of willpower, since the girl is presented as unable to "break away from this guy." The verb phrase "break away" expresses quite a violent notion of separating oneself from another person, and it therefore appears in stark contrast to the depiction of the girl as weak both in physique and in character. Moreover, the verb metaphorically implies a unity between the boyfriend and the girl that can only be disrupted by means of forceful action. Thus, the GP implicitly establishes a causal link between the girl's weakness and the fact that "she just couldn't do anything about it" (line 6).

The doctor's own helplessness is expressed in the conditional clause in line 7, "no matter what we suggested," and in the evaluative clause in line 4, "that was really sad," where the intensifier "really" again stresses the GP's emotional judgment. Interestingly enough, the GP uses the fact that the girl did not leave her partner as a means of classifying her as "different." In other words, the GP implies that other victims of domestic abuse normally manage to escape the violence. This might hint at the GP's misconception of violent relationships, which are often of longer duration and might involve continued violence even after the woman has left her partner (Schornstein 1997:26). It is also noteworthy that the GP presents the domestic violence case against a background of drug-taking and criminal activities. A common cliché is drawn upon and at the same time reinforced (see chapter 6).

The GP's Expression of Her Limited View of the Patient in Narrative 11

Narrative 11 is marked by a lengthy complicating action sequence, which ranges from line 5 to line 11. One would expect an end in line 6, the end either of the girl's embedded story (she was abused) or of the GP's framing story (she realized that the girl was being abused). However, the end is elided in favor of listing a number of subsequent events. In other words, the story never comes to an end, thereby beginning to clarify why doctors do not do well with domestic violence cases. Many of the narratives in my sample are similarly narratologically complicated. The use of the past progressive form in line 5 ("and she was coming in with . . .") indicates that the girl must have come regularly within a certain period of time that is not further specified. The signs of violence are fairly obvious: black eyes, bruises, and "all sorts of things" (line 5). The description also becomes vague through the less specified noun phrase. Line 9 is significant in the narration, as it interrupts the continuity of this girl's story of recurrent injuries and repeat visits to the health center. The girl was "much better" while her boyfriend was in prison, that is, while she was not exposed to his violence. This clause almost appears as a ray of hope in the GP's narrative, and it can be seen as equivalent to a delaying factor in the development of this tragic story.

The allusion to the overall structure of tragedies seems adequate in this context if we consider the remainder of the complicating action sequence in lines 10 and 11: "and she just, she didn't finish her degree and she just looked iller and iller and more and more tired." The negator in "she didn't finish her degree" (line 10) and the combination of the repeated comparators "iller and iller" and "more and more tired" mark the gradual but definite physical decline of this girl and thus her overall downfall, which can be interpreted as a *falling action*. The *catastrophe*, however, is not fully borne out, since the ending is left open: the GP does not know "what's happened" to the girl (line 13) because the girl "just disappeared" (line 12). In a sense, the girl's bodily consumption culminates in her physical disappearance.

The clause in line 15 functions as a coda and ties the action of the narrative back to the present. At this point the GP states that "goodness knows where she is now." The formulaic expression "goodness knows" implies in an almost fatalistic tone that it cannot possibly be in the GP's power to know what happened to the girl or where she is located at present. The conjunction "where," indicating place or, in this case, a lack of spatial orientation, reveals the limitation of the "medical gaze": if patients do not come to the GPs to present their problems, there is no way for GPs to know what else is going on in patients' lives, and doctors do not even feel it is their place to do anything about patients' problems. One young female GP commented:

> 1. But part of me also makes me think, and **it's perhaps unfair,** but part of me makes me think that I wish women had the confidence and tell us if there was a problem. . . . It's **hard enough to do** anyway but **we're not mind readers** and if we're having a busy surgery and **all we see is the pink page in front of us.** We're not looking through notes all the time and analyzing everybody's consultation. So, if they come in with a sore throat we deal with their sore throat and then they go but if they just gave us some, some better clues.

What strikes one immediately in this passage is the GP's reluctance to appear critical of patients. The hedge "it's perhaps unfair" and also the noun phrase "part of me" indicate that the GP is not entirely sure whether her statement will be interpreted by the interviewer as unjust criticism and therefore requires mitigation. These features illustrate the validity of the theoretical proposition that discourse is always socially situated and that speakers accommodate linguistically to each other by means of word choice, for example. At the same time, one of the assumptions I made in chapter 3 is borne out by the data, namely, that defensive answers might indicate that the GP felt threatened by potential criticism on the part of the interviewer.

This doctor, like most of the female GPs in the sample, is fairly open in admitting that it is difficult to deal with domestic violence. By using the image of the "mind readers" she depicts domestic violence as something obscure that can only be revealed in a paranormal or supernatural way unless the patients give "some better clues." Patients become equivalent to the "pink page" in front of the doctor, that is, they are reduced to a fact sheet that presents in a very abbreviated and specially encoded way the patient's history of illness. The consultation is depicted as an event limited both in time and space. The doctor not only has little time available during a "busy surgery," but he or she also lacks the time to look through notes and to investigate a patient's case history more holistically. The case as such is in turn confined to the "pink sheet" of the medical record. The only way domestic violence can be discovered in such a restricted context, it seems, is by means of very obvious external evidence in terms of physical signs of abuse. Otherwise, as one late-middle-aged male GP pointed out, "there is no magic way of finding it out." The same GP expanded on the mental image of magic by conjuring up a whole consultation scenario with a touch of science fiction attached to it:

> 2. Um, sometimes it's very well **hidden.** Now, should I be expected to have **x-ray specs** to be able to in all cases find, er, each and every case? It depends on **degree** I think. I, we can't, we know, we're, we're **general practice specialists** but, um, we do not have, um, some **magic scanner that comes** [**on over the door**] **with flashes** when somebody's undergoing, er, abuse. Er, I think we are well placed to **discover** it when it's at a **level** which does become **obvious.**

Domestic violence is depicted as something that is "hidden" and that GPs can only "discover" when it is "obvious." The impossibility of finding out about it in all other cases is dramatized in the futuristic image of the "x-ray specs" and the "magic scanner." By using this highly technical imagery the GP implicitly points out medicine's inadequacy in dealing with problems that do not follow the biomedical model and that can therefore not be discovered by means of medical apparatus. After all, high technology is "the epitome of the 'biomedical model,'" as Annandale (1998:271) maintains.

Another interesting feature in this passage is the GP's mentioning of a "degree" or "level" of violence, thus assuming that violence is gradable in terms of severity. This is a line of reasoning that appears frequently in the GPs' discourses. Doctors conceptualized domestic abuse as a "continuum" that could thus be dealt with "on different levels." In other words, the severity of the violence displayed to the doctor has an impact on the GP's reaction and subsequent provision of salient help. In the excerpt above the message is fairly straightforward: unless domestic violence is "obvious," visible as marks or bruisings, the GP cannot discover it. As one middle-aged female GP remarked, "it's almost got to be in your face." These comments indicate that GPs possibly lack sensitivity to subtler signs of abuse or that they tend to overlook problems that do not "fit the medical wardrobe," as one female GP put it metaphorically. While there is at first glance nothing wrong with physicians dealing primarily with physical symptoms, a problem arises when doctors focus so much on the physical side of things that they overlook other possible signs and miss a diagnosis, as I discussed in the previous chapter. Moreover, doctors' immersion in the biomedical model can be detrimental if it causes them to deny their responsibility in "nonmedical" problems. A number of GPs in my sample emphasized that they did not think it was their place to do anything about domestic violence, since it was primarily a social problem. (This particular explanation is explored further in the next chapter.) That GPs are sometimes quite remote from their patients' lives and their problems not only spatially but perhaps also conceptually can be seen in the way the GPs spoke about their work and the practice environment.

Path Schema
One metaphoric category that pervades the GPs' narratives is the *path* schema. As I mentioned above, paths are important, since they connect the spatial world around us. As Johnson points out, the "PATH schema is one of the most common structures that emerges from our constant bodily functioning" (1987:116),

and it therefore serves as a basis for a number of metaphors: "In our culture, for example, we have a metaphorical understanding of the passage of time based on movement along a physical path. We understand mental activities or operations that result in some determinate outcome according to the PATH schema. And we understand the course of processes in general metaphorically as movement along a path toward some end point" (1987:117). The GPs in my sample regularly used spatial language in order to depict the way they would try to find out more about underlying issues or, once domestic abuse has been established, what their next steps would be. To see how the path schema is borne out in the GPs' responses, consider the following examples:

3. a. I think it would be a case of **flying by the seat of your pants,** see what kind of reaction you're getting and, er, **exploring** this more.

b. You're obliged to ask how things are at home and to **follow that avenue** in addition to what's happening at work, financial pressures, and all the other pressures that are on us today.

c. I suppose you have to **backtrack** really and see what their pattern of consultation has been and what exactly they're coming along with.

d. In a sort of **roundabout way,** I suppose, that's what we're really asking.

e. We probably don't **go out** [**of our way**] because we know, we know it's a **difficult area,** we don't feel we can do much.

f. There are difficulties with culture, with admitting to, to depression and other kinds of mental illness and it causes offense to ask these questions whereas it doesn't cause offense to, to **go down the physical route.**

4. a. I sympathized with her, I **sent her on her way.**

b. Even if it's just a few girls that we **could set off in the right direction,** give them a fresh start it'd be worth it.

c. I still think, at the end of the day, that the, the person who is being victimized has to **make the first step.** I don't think people can do it for them. If they're willing to just accept it, that is, as I say, hard luck. They just have to be prepared to **go forward** and get help.

d. You can't really stop them and say: "Look, this isn't my problem. Go to a social worker!" If you do that you're not gonna do them any favors 'cause it might be the only, the one and only time that they've spoken to somebody about it. To **stop them in their tracks** at that point really wouldn't be any good.

e. You have to hope that if they're coming then they actually are looking to **find a way through** to talk about it.

f. I think, if, er, if they've got information about **places that they could go** so then, even if they **go home** to the same situation and do nothing, if they've got those numbers, should it recur or should there be a crisis then at least they feel they've got a safety net or they've got an **escape route.**

What strikes one immediately in these responses is the fact that GPs conceptualize different paths for patients and for themselves in their cognitive mappings. The answers in (3) represent paths taken by GPs in their practice work, while the answers in (4) illustrate the paths GPs envisage for their patients. Thus, doctors can take the "physical route" in a consultation, that is, examine a patient merely with regard to physical problems, or they can follow the route of asking more private questions and "fly by the seat of their pants" in order to discover more hidden issues. In other words, GPs can rely on their experience in certain cases. Interestingly enough, the option of flying by the seat of one's pants in (3a) is introduced in the hypothetical mode through the modal auxiliary "would" and is thus indirectly presented as a rather unusual option for GPs.[2] This could be related to the fact that GPs perceive cases of domestic violence as infrequent in their practices, or it might point toward doctors' reluctance to ask questions concerning violence. As the GP in (3e) admits, "we probably don't go out of our way" because domestic violence is a "difficult area" and thus potentially dangerous.

The notion of danger as well as of adventure and risk taking is evoked not only through the verb phrases that construct paths for the GPs ("flying," "explore," and "go out of our way") but also through the mentioning of the "escape route" that women can access once they have obtained sufficient information on "places that they could go" (4f). This imagery indicates GPs' conceptualization of domestic violence as "dangerous ground" that they might wish to avoid. One way of doing this is to disentangle mentally the spatial networks of doctors and patients and to pass the responsibility of finding appropriate paths onto the woman. Thus, GPs can set patients "off in the right direction" (4b), but, ultimately, the victim is "on *her* way" (4a, my emphasis), and she has to "go forward and get help," as the GP in (4c) put it bluntly. Victims of domestic violence have to "find a way through" (4e) to their GP, which again implies a distance between doctors and patients, as the "way" or "path" described is not one that the GP equally enters and follows. By linguistically creating different "route maps" for their patients and for themselves, GPs reinforce the spatial distance that is already in place through the layout of the consultation room, which is secluded from the life world of the patient.

Mapping out the Consultation

Although GPs also conduct house calls, their normal workplace is the practice and, within the practice, the consultation room of each individual doctor. Patients usually go to the practice to present their problems, and both the examination of the patient and the GP's diagnosis as well as the initiation of treatment take place within the confined space of the consultation room. In other words, the location of medical interviews is relatively fixed, and the doctor as one actor in this setting is also a more or less stationary "object" in this spatial environment. The patient, on the other hand, appears as a variable and mobile actor:

> 5. a. There's a lot of domestic disharmony, er, and on occasions people will **come along** with stories of, well, physical violence or mental violence, mostly mental, I think.
>
> b. Occasionally people **come in** and present their, their bruises.
>
> c. When they **come in the door** they've decided what they're going to say.

d. I certainly do have a lot of depressed patients **coming**, um, **through my doors.**

e. Unless they see it as a medical problem they're not probably gonna **walk through the door** with that.

f. It may be that the woman **turns up at the surgery** with an appointment, er, either on an urgent basis or as part of a routine appointment, and will usually in the course of the consultation say that she wants to, um, confide that she's been abused.

g. If you're a doctor you have to give it high priority in your surgery but, I mean, you're **not in control** of that. You **don't know what's coming in that door.** Somebody **comes in the door** and [might] have a stroke **in front of you,** that's not going to take half an hour, it's not, y——, you've got no control of that.

The spatiotemporal map that is created in these examples is based on two spatial vectors: one mobile vector, whereby the patient "comes in that door" (5g), and one static vector, which indicates what happens "in front of" the doctor. Temporally, the incident is unpredictable, that is, it can happen anytime in any consultation, and it clearly disrupts the flow of the consultation and, ultimately, of the entire appointment schedule.

"Come" is by far the most commonly used motion verb in the GPS' discourse, and it is normally combined with the spatial adverbs "in" or "along" to delineate the patients' movements. Significantly enough, "come" in narratives presents movement of a person other than the speaker from a farther removed place toward the speaker: "*come, arrive, walk in* are used of entry into the space (corridor, room or office) which is nearest to the observer in each episode" (Brown 1995:190). In the doctors' responses the point of view taken up is the one of the GP, who is located at the center both of the practice environment and of the narrative concerning the encounter with a patient during a consultation. In addition, the locatives "in" (5b), "in the door" (5c), "through my doors" (5d), and "through the door" (5e) create a mental image of the practice as an enclosed place, as they evoke the *container metaphor* (Lakoff and Johnson 1980). The practice is envisaged as a kind of "container" with an opening, the door, through which patients move in and out. The following comment made by a middle-aged male GP illustrates the perception of patients "passing by" through the practice:

> 6. It's not something that you see every week or every month. Some-times you see it, **it's like buses,** you know, [they] **come along,** you know. . . . Um, I mean it's **rare for it to be declared.** You know, it's **not common** for women to **come in and say, you know:** "**I'm suf-fering.**" Er, it's generally **uncovered** in, in other ways.

The simile "like buses" refers to the folk saying that they come all at once or not at all. It draws upon the image of movement of one object (bus, patient) rela-tive to a person (traveler, doctor). By equating himself with a traveler waiting for a bus, the GP implicitly defines his own role as passive and thus limited. He himself does not move anywhere but waits in his practice for patients to "come along." At the same time, domestic violence is presented as something the doc-tor does not encounter very often in patients. The tautology of "rare" and "not common" emphasizes the infrequency of disclosures of domestic abuse, which is depicted twice in this comment: first, through the passive infinitive construc-tion "to be declared," and second, through the active construction whereby "women come in and say, you know, 'I'm suffering.'" The active role of the pa-tient is stressed by direct speech. Ironically, however, this active part is already negated by the doctor's statement that this type of disclosure is rare. Another interesting feature in this comment is the past participle "uncovered," which conveys an image of domestic violence as being something hidden.

Spatiotemporal Mapping and the (Re)Construction of Domestic Violence as a "Hidden" Problem

The estimated frequency of visits by patients who suffer domestic abuse varies considerably in the interviews. Variations in the responses sometimes occurred even in interviews conducted within the same practice. Few doctors were able to quantify their encounters with domestic violence victims, and among those who provided a figure, it ranged from "one or two a fortnight" over "one a month" to "two or three times a year." One young male GP stated that he had never had a case of domestic violence in the practice that he was working in at the time of the interview, and a middle-aged female GP said that she could "count on one hand" all the cases she had ever encountered. Interestingly enough, this female GP worked in a practice with patients from mainly deprived social backgrounds. Moreover, another GP from the same practice who had been interviewed in the first round of pilot interviews had stated that he frequently saw patients suffering domestic violence. Does this contradiction indicate that the female GP is possibly unable to detect the problem? Likewise, out of three GPs who worked in the same health center two (young, male and female) stated that they saw domestic violence frequently in their patients, while the third middle-aged female GP said that she did not encounter it as regularly as she had done when she worked in Edinburgh in the 1980s. The discrepancy in these GPs' responses shows that GPs may perceive the frequency of domestic violence cases differently, depending on previous work experience with this problem. If the third doctor, however, indeed encountered fewer patients who suffer domestic violence than her colleagues despite the fact that they all work within the same practice population, then questions arise as to whether this may have to do with less awareness of or receptiveness to the problem.

We cannot necessarily generalize by correlating the occurrence of domestic abuse with lower social status. However, the interviews revealed a tendency of GPs working in socially deprived areas to be, on the whole, more aware of domestic violence in their patients. One explanation might be that domestic violence is disclosed more frequently by patients from lower social backgrounds, while middle-class patients are more strongly inhibited by the social stigma attached to domestic abuse. As one male GP nearing retirement observed, "they don't bother to cover up in the same way as do the more affluent areas." It is equally plausible, however, that GPs do not expect domestic violence in middle-class patients and therefore fail to notice indirect signs of abuse such as depression, nervous conditions, sleeplessness, and fatigue. This indicates that the disclosure of domestic violence depends on GPs' perceptions and on whether they are alert to underlying issues or not rather than on the socioeconomic status of the practice population.

Most of the GPs in my sample said that domestic violence was not something they encountered very often, and GPs regularly admitted that a lot more might be going on without them being aware of it. The following responses illustrate this awareness:

7. a. I'm probably aware statistically [that] there's **a lot more goes on** but, er, there's, er, there's not all that, in the course of a year, **not all that many get positively brought to our attention.**

b. We know from research that **it is a lot more common than we usually pick up.** . . . So we also know there is a huge number of, um, there are **a huge number of women out there** who probably experience domestic violence.

c. I'm not, **not a lot is disclosed to you.**

d. Not much, to be honest, um, or **people don't approach me** particularly.

e. I think there's **an awful lot underlying that we never really broach.**

f. I mean there's times where you're, you're almost certain that it is, that they, the woman won't admit it or you have a hunch but they don't want to talk about it and they, you know, they'll, they'll cov—
—, **they'll cover it up,** and other times, I'm absolutely positive, **we don't think about it.**

g. I'm trying to see it **from their perspective,** that they have **come** and they may **find the door shut.** They expect us to **try and open the door and we didn't.** And then they may then go back into their old situation and go, "There's nae point in going to see the [doctor] because . . ." you know [clears his throat]

h. I think there's a hidden, **huge hidden,** you know, **mass of it** that **no one comes forward**

The spatiotemporal language in these comments reveals a number of expectations and visualizations. First of all, domestic violence is presented as a problem that appears to be more frequent than GPs recognize in their practice work. Furthermore, domestic violence is presented as "hidden" (7h) and as an "underlying" (7e) problem that patients "cover up" (7f). The spatial position of domestic violence is thus defined as "low," "on the ground," or even "underground," which can also be seen in the frequently occurring verb phrase "pick it up" (7b). The vector representing movement in this mental image reaches from the ground upward and thus locates the object to be picked up on ground level.[3] GPs described domestic violence as a "bottomless pit," the "root problems" of which they could not solve. Cases "bubbled up on the surface" in "oblique presentations," which makes it particularly difficult for GPs to bring them out "into the open." GPs are also often not prepared to "dig deeper in a dodgy clinical history," as one young male GP put it, drawing upon the pit image. One late-middle-aged male GP cynically contended that domestic violence "gets just swept under the carpet by everybody. The perpetrator, the victim, the doctor, the police, everybody." The reason this GP offered for the kind of active and collective neglect of domestic abuse includes people's unwillingness to assume responsibility: "Because, if you can't quantify it and if you can't qualify it and you can't be certain that it's happening how can you do anything about it?" Despite this open critique, the same GP continued by justifying GPs' behavior, stating that it was "beyond the GP's role" to deal with domestic violence in the limited consultation time. The preposition "beyond" creates a further spatial image with regard to domestic violence cases. Domestic violence is not only "low" and "underground" but also spatially removed from the GP's sphere of activity and responsibilities.

Spatiotemporal Limitations and GPs' Explanations for the Nondetection of Domestic Violence

Another spatial relationship depicted in the GPs' responses is the one between doctor and patient. Example (7b) is interesting in this respect because it creates an image of a divide between patients and their doctors: there are a lot of "women *out there* who probably experience domestic violence." Significantly enough, women who suffer abuse are not located inside the practice. In other words, this GP implicitly recognizes the absence of domestic violence in the secluded environment of the practice. What also features very strongly in the GPs' responses is their expectation that the patient discloses her problem, as can be seen in (7a), (7c), and (7d). GPs seem to expect patients to "approach" them or to "bring" problems to their attention, and if patients fail to do so, doctors "never really broach" (7e) certain issues. As the middle-aged male GP in (7g) comments, patients might also come with certain expectations and sometimes find the "door shut" because the GP failed to "open the door." The door and gatekeeping metaphor again evokes a sense of distance and separation between doctor and patient, but this time the blame for this separation is put on the GP.

Response (7g) is particularly interesting, as it reveals the culture specificity of people's expectations and their linguistic renditions. The "open door" metaphor relates to the Western notion of an "open door policy," for example, which involves receptiveness, readiness to be helpful, and so on. This kind of behavior may be expected by patients who are hoping to disclose their problems to their GP. On the other hand, the image of "closed doors" also has to do with notions of privacy and prohibitions to trespass on other people's private spheres. This is the view GPs might adopt when they do not wish to interfere with their patients' private lives. The door metaphor itself thus creates problems through its polysemy, which may lead to concrete difficulties in doctor-patient interaction. The relative frequency of this image in the GPs' responses, however, indicates that it belongs to a cognitive framework by which GPs rationalize their relationships with their patients.

The reasons that emerge for nondisclosure and nondetection of domestic violence are twofold: on the one hand, doctors tend to expect patients to play a more active role and to open up; on the other hand, GPs themselves often deliberately refrain from broaching the subject with patients for reasons of time, stress, or fear of emotional involvement.

Spatiotemporal Mapping, Metaphors, and the Threat to the "Ceremonial Order" in Medical Consultations

When doctors and patients meet they automatically assume their roles in what Strong calls the "bureaucratic role format" of medical encounters, which comprises, among other elements, doctors' authority over patients and control of the interaction as well as a heavily routinized speech style that allows only little information to be imparted to patients and that affords them only few opportunities to express their own views (1979:9, 199–200). This bureaucratic role format by necessity involves the negotiation of identities, and identities, in turn, incorporate moral status, as Strong emphasizes:

Identity is the central topic on which any ceremonial order legis-
lates, and moral status is a fundamental part of that identity. But
since the ceremonial order is a matter of outward show, the moral
order which it creates is regularly threatened by the actual facts of
the case and by the incidents and upsets that occur in any form of
human intercourse. In consequence, the parties to an encounter
are presented with a series of constant challenges, either actual or
potential, which threaten their moral worth or that of their fellow
participants. (1979:41)

Domestic violence poses a threat to the ritual "ceremonial order" of medical
encounters, according to which the encounter "normally" takes place smoothly
and without major disturbances. It frequently comes out somewhat unexpect-
edly for the doctor, and it also involves questions of confidentiality, responsibility, and agency. Put another way, domestic violence is something that doctors
do not feel in control of once it comes to the surface. This threat is linguistically
conceptualized in the "tip of the iceberg" and the "can of worms" metaphors,
for example, by which GPs implicitly express their fears and anxieties.

Metaphors Expressing Doctors' Anxiety
The Journey Metaphor
One metaphor that can be regarded as a subcategory of the path schema is the
journey metaphor. This metaphor has been internalized by speakers of English to such an extent that it is often no longer conspicuous, as Lakoff (1993)
emphasizes in his discussion of the *love-is-a-journey metaphor*. Since the journey image is such an internalized concept, however, it is worthwhile analyzing
the cognitive mapping that underlies this metaphor in the GPs' narrative discourse. One young male GP stated, for example, that "GPs are the most likely
first port of call" for patients who suffer domestic violence, that is, the practice
is the place where patients expect to end their often long "journey" of suffering.
While this metaphor potentially opens vistas for lengthy life stories, the narratives of the GPs often refer to but rarely elaborate on the patient's "life journey." In a sense, the metaphor thus becomes a substitute for fully fledged, temporally extended narratives.

Patients' suffering is often described by doctors as part of a many-faceted
picture of misery, as in the following explanation for the occurrence of domestic violence provided by a middle-aged female GP:

8. You have to go round some of the areas in Aberdeen to see these houses and think, well, you know, if you're **trooped up** with three kids in a room with no carpets and, you know, you've got into a habit of drug abuse, say, but, you know, the tensions must be absolutely awful if there's, if there seems to be **no future** for people, which, I think, is often in the deprived areas, that seems to be the major thing, there's no jobs, the housing's poor, everyone is [?] **in the same boat.**

Domestic violence is correlated with a low socioeconomic background and poor living conditions, and these factors are captured in the military imagery present in the predicative adjective "trooped up" and the voyage metaphor that envisages all these people "in the same boat."[4] *Life is a journey* is the underlying metaphor in this mental image. The journey metaphor, however, is also used in the more specific context of the consultation, as the following response shows:

9. Um, and, you know, a lot of them will, um, be just [waiting] to see if you're gonna be receptive to what they're saying and they'll, they'll give you a few minutes to see if you're listening and then they'll tell you what they're really here for. And I think you have to sort of **take that on board.**

Here, the consultation is indirectly mapped onto the image of a voyage during which specific facets of the consultation and the patient's behavior can be "taken on board," that is, considered, by the GP. This metaphor, although it will be understood by most speakers of English, also avoids an exact statement of how this action is undertaken. In other words, the metaphor abbreviates a longer narrative of "how" the patient's behavior can be "taken on board" by the doctor. The concept, and thus perhaps also its underlying practice, remains vague and opaque.

The Iceberg Metaphor
Another metaphor that five of the twenty GPs used was that of the iceberg. Domestic violence is equated with an iceberg, and the common denominators for this equation are size and the fact that the largest part of the mass remains underwater. Put another way, the problem of domestic abuse is conceptualized as a "huge" problem, but it is also a problem of which doctors see only the small part that is brought out into the open. Consider the following examples:

10. a. So it's, it's, so this is, there's a **huge mountain** of, you know, it's like an iceberg. Whether there's a whole lot of people **under the surface** there that just don't speak about it at all, you don't hear about it, er, I really don't know.

b. I mean, we only probably see the **tip of the iceberg** though, um, sort of stressed, depressed people who if you sort of **enquire** a bit further, you **discover** that there's a bit of it going on.

c. It's quite a **horrible thought** to think that we are probably **missing** a lot of it but I'm sure there must be, you know, it must, it must just be the **tip of the iceberg** what we're seeing.

Domestic violence cases are visualized as an amorphous lump rather than as a quantifiable medical problem, and this image is primarily used by the GPs to explain why they probably miss so much of it, namely, because the problem is not easily quantifiable and thus not identifiable, or vice versa, and because it remains secret, opaque, and hidden in most cases. The iceberg metaphor also carries undertones of fear and helplessness. Icebergs are commonly considered dangerous exactly because there is this huge hidden mass under the water that can destroy ships even when they seem to be far away from the tip of the iceberg. Bearing this additional facet in mind, GPs' reference to the iceberg metaphor in their narratives can also be interpreted as an indirect expression of their feeling of being threatened by a problem that they are inadequately equipped to deal with. In a similar vein, one male GP commented: "It's too big a, er, it's too big a job to, to take on board, er, personal issues from people," thereby evoking the journey metaphor, albeit in negative terms. And a female GP described her decision as to whether to broach the issue with a patient or not in the following way:

11. It can depend entirely on how relaxed you feel like, you know, if you don't feel there's any pressure to get this surgery [appointment] finished on time or whatever else, then those are the days when you may well decide to **dip the toe in the water** or the, the, you know, sometimes it's just not possible.

The image used here clearly emphasizes GPs' hesitant behavior when it comes to dealing with emotional problems in their patients.

Opening up a Can of Worms

One phrase that six of the GPs used to explain why they often deliberately refrained from broaching the issue of domestic violence with patients is "opening up a can of worms." By using this metaphor doctors implied not only that the problem of domestic abuse might not be closed again once it was opened up but also that it is difficult to control because it might branch out into various directions. The following responses reveal this concern:

> 12. a. Um, you certainly can **detect** that there might be **a can of worms** there, and you then have a **choice of whether to open the can or not open the can.** And I think, as a doctor, you, you, you may [have to] follow your judgment sometimes.
>
> b. We're **overwhelmed** by people's physi——, physical problems and mental problems. Trying to deal with social problems as well, you know, is, is just, yeah, it's probably **easier not to ask that question,** to open that can of worms **in a lot of cases.**
>
> c. I mean if, if it's been going on for ages, er, and I know that it would be **a can of worms** that would be opened, **I will maybe leave it.**
>
> d. There's a bit of a **fear about bringing things out into the open** as well 'cause [that] can **open up a huge can of worms** and, and that probably, you know, we probably save our time in the long run if we were to bring this out into the open because a lot of these girls I'm sure are coming along with minor complaints and, you know, some things that we can't ex——, can't perhaps explain and there is domestic violence **underlying** all of this so, in the long run, we might save ourselves appointments but sometimes you're **scared just to open up that can of worms** 'cause often I don't know, **I don't feel there's an awful lot practical we can do** to support them.

e. What I as a GP have got to offer is, I guess, quite limited. [They might sort of think that] can be **opening a can of worms that I can't deal with.**

f. Um, and a lot of it is, I think, I think they feel that [if] they speak to their GP they're **opening a can of worms and that it can't be closed again** and what do they do after that?

A can of worms evokes associations with uncontrollability and also with a notion of ugliness of the issue. Worms are considered to be unpleasant or a nuisance and are thus something that people would rather not have to deal with. Similarly, domestic violence can contain a number of other unpleasant issues, not least the patient's distress in that situation. The container metaphor is drawn upon in this image, but this time the container is not empty like the "bottomless pit" mentioned above. Instead, the container is full of "ugly" problems and further difficulties that are uncontrollable. Once the worms are out of the can they cannot be put back into it. Consequently, GPs feel "scared" (12d) to open this can of worms because they are already "overwhelmed" by people's "physical" and "mental," in other words, medical, problems (12b). The metaphors and spatiotemporal expressions used by the GPs reveal their mental "visualizations" of domestic violence cases and point toward underlying concerns and anxieties. Due to these anxieties doctors may well decide not to broach the issue with a patient even if they have a suspicion that something else is going on. They have "the choice of whether to open the can or not open the can," as the GP in (12a) put it in a Hamletish manner, and very often they decide to just "leave it" (12a) and "not to ask that question" (12b). In other words, whether disclosure takes place within a consultation also depends very much on GPs' judgment and on their decision about whether they want to uncover things or not. GPs can either pass over the issue altogether, whether deliberately or unintentionally, in order to decrease the disrupting effect of disclosure or they can attempt to formalize the situation and make it more "orderly," as it were, by following the "paths" currently available in general practice, which mainly involve treatment of physical injuries and onward referral to other agencies. In (12e) and (12f) the doctors attempt to adopt their patients' point of view by stating that disclosure can mean opening a can of worms for victims, too, especially if they think that the GP cannot really help them further. This view, however, especially if it becomes part of doctors' "storied knowledge," only perpetuates GPs' belief that they are ill equipped to deal with domestic abuse, which might ultimately influence their practice work and thus also be reflected in their patients' reactions to them.

Methodically, the analysis of the GPs' linguistic representation of "space-time regions" in their narratives shows how microstructural and macrolevel approaches can be combined: the GPs' discursive strategy of distancing reveals and also reinforces their conceptual separation of their own, that is, medical, space from their patients' personal space, on which domestic violence has an impact.[5] This distance can also be seen in GPs' linguistic "visualizations" of backgrounds to domestic violence situations, which I discuss in the next chapter. While the focus in this chapter lay on metaphors, including spatiotemporal frameworks, the next chapter expands on this discussion by investigating the ways in which GPs use such conceptual frameworks in order to mythologize both their own work conditions and backgrounds and scenarios of abuse. I demonstrate that the myths thus created serve as explanations and excuses for doctors' seemingly limited scope of action with regard to domestic violence cases.

6. Mythologizing Time, Mythologizing Violence
Backgrounds and Explanations of Domestic Abuse

If we follow the pioneering work of structural anthropologist Lévi-Strauss (1986), we can conceive of myths as cognitive devices, as ways of organizing and understanding reality in a given cultural context. In his *Mythologies* Barthes (1972) defines myths as secondary semiotic systems that mystify reality and that people are made to believe. Myths are steeped in a culture's beliefs and values. To give a very simple example, the specific shape and horsepower of a particular brand of car signifies that car owner's economic power and social status. In everyday myths a second reality is constructed and naturalized. The strength of myths lies in their ability to cater to the "need for a single, comprehensive account" (Spence 1998:221). As Spence points out, the "mythic explanation, as it feeds on other popular accounts, tends to suppress complicating variations and replace them with a kind of uniform simplicity" (1998:221). Myths are created to be integrated into certain organizational discourses, in this particular case the discourse of the medical profession, that in turn help establish and sustain power relationships (Fairclough 1989, 2001). In chapter 3 I listed a number of myths surrounding the problem of domestic violence. In this chapter I investigate in what ways the GPs' narratives also perpetuate such common myths and to what extent this may have an influence on how doctors perceive their own role as health care professionals who have to deal with this problem. The constitutive nature of GPs' discourse thus becomes a crucial question and requires further exploration in my narrative analyses. While sociological studies have concentrated on the surface realizations of myths and stereotypes in social discourses, this study goes a step further and uncovers the linguistic mechanisms in operation that create such myths in the GPs' discourse. I commence this chapter with a discussion of time as a recurring theme in the GPs' narratives, thereby tying back to my investigation of spatiotemporal mapping in the previous chapter.

Mythologizing Time in General Practice

Time invariably flared up as a topic during the interviews and in the GPs' narratives. On the one hand, the doctors viewed time with regard to the patient, who often suffers domestic violence over a lengthy period of time. Below I discuss cycle-of-abuse theories and family histories of violence as explanatory frameworks in the GPs' narratives. On the other hand, the doctors related time to general practice and health care and to their own job and training as general practitioners. The impact of "clock time" on the consultation can in turn be viewed from two perspectives. First, patients are not granted enough time to elaborate their possibly complex self-narratives; and second, doctors do not have the opportunity to explore their patients holistically and consequently fail to create a "medical narrative" with sufficiently detailed information. Instead, their rather schematized medical record may well lack clues to adequate treatment. As a study on decision making and consent to treatment in general surgery has shown, doctors' lack of time very often hinders successful interaction and communication between doctor and patient (Meredith 1993). The same result has been found for consultations on domestic violence (Sugg and Inui 1992). Warshaw's (1993) study on the treatment of battered women in an urban emergency room demonstrates that time constraints linked up with overwork and understaffing led to nondetection and nonintervention and, more important, to a lack of response and receptiveness by nurses and doctors. I would argue that GPs' tendency to use medical "shorthand" rather than complex narrative in medical examinations precludes the emergence of holistic patient stories with salient hints at possible underlying problems. Moreover, as I discussed in the previous chapter, time pressure coupled with the emotional and psychological demands of dealing with domestic violence cases may lead to anxieties.

One young female GP in my sample considered time such an important factor that it even became the topic of a lengthy narrative. Narrative 28 was related in the context of a discussion of time with regard to the problem of asking patients about domestic violence. The GP maintained that, in spite of time constraints, she "would tend to ask them anyway." The narrative, however, illustrates the problem of time pressure in a consultation.

Narrative 28

1. I had one girl who, ach, she had a horrible family.[1]
2. She, her, her mother told her when she was, ach I don't know, just

     about eighteen, that her father wasn't her father and "by the way, that's your father over there."

3. And so she'd become very confused
4. and I tried to approach him
5. and then, a year or so later, the mother said: "Now, that was all a lie, he's not your father at all, blah blah blah"
6. and there was a whole big [discussion] about the families
7. and she was very upset about it.
8. You know, she was dressed,
9. she set to work, when you actually went into it,
10. and you really had to go into that in detail,
11. but I said to her: "Well, you know, we've cer——, I've [been] speaking for about twenty minutes. [I'm kind of] running out of time."
12. So, get her to come back
13. and some will come back, some won't.
14. She did come back
15. but, um, you do have to give them the chance to say it.

Time Constraints as "Reportable"
Narrative Topic: Analysis of Narrative 28

The narrative is interesting, as two stories intermingle in it: the one of the patient's family and the story about the consultation during which the patient revealed her family background to the doctor. What strikes us about this story is its confusion and lack of more detailed information. The GP tells the interviewer how the girl found out about her father, and she does it by combining indirect and direct discourse: "her mother told her when she was, ach I don't know, just about eighteen, that her father wasn't her father and 'by the way, that's your father over there'" (line 2). In switching from a report of the mother's speech to a direct representation of it, which also involves a shift in deictic features such as the personal pronoun "you" and the locative "over there," the GP discursively brings the scene to life as it probably occurred between mother and daughter. A similar strategy is adopted in line 5, where the GP again "quotes" directly what the mother said. The GP even goes as far as to mock the mother's talk by presenting it as general blabber: "That was all a lie, he's not your father at all, blah blah blah" (line 5). On the one hand, this ridicules and downgrades the mother; on the other hand, it abbreviates the narrative. Thus, the information given remains rather incomplete and causes the listener to be as confused as the patient in that situation.

Lines 6 and 7 again summarize in very brief terms what happened after this disclosure and how it affected the patient: "and there was a whole big [discussion] about the families and she was very upset about it." Part of the confusion created in this narrative can be attributed to the fact that the GP uses an elliptical time frame to relate the story. Thus, for example, there is a gap between the time the patient hears for the first time about the family situation—"she was, ach I don't know, just about eighteen" (line 2)—and the time when her mother negates her previous statement—"then, a year or so later, the mother said" (line 5). The only two snippets of information concerning the interim period relate to the patient's reaction and the fact that the GP attempted to mediate between her and the alleged father: "And so she'd become very confused and I tried to approach him" (lines 3–4). The sequential order of these events is indicated by the consequential coordinators "and so" as well as the order of the clauses. Generally speaking, the narrative remains rather skeletal, as it does not provide any further information on what exactly the background to this strange family situation was or why the mother lied to her daughter. More important, the GP does not even clarify whether there was any domestic violence at stake, which, after all, was the main topic of the interview.

The reason for this brevity becomes obvious in the second part of the story, when the GP moves toward the actual point of the narrative, namely, her lack of time in the consultation with this particular patient. The clauses in lines 8 and 9 seem to be misplaced at first glance, as they also provide general information and thus belong to the orientation: "You know, she was dressed, she set to work, when you actually went into it." The discourse marker "you know," by contrasting with the conjunction "and," which started the five preceding clauses, introduces a new topic: the way the patient was perceived by the doctor during the consultation. The family history can thus be recognized in retrospect as a preliminary story that was probably related by the patient during the consultation. Put another way, the GP relates in her narrative a story that had been told in yet another storytelling situation: the consultation. At the same time, the GP defines her own role in that storytelling situation as "going into it," that is, trying to gain more information from the patient: "and you really had to go into that in detail" (line 10). Thus, the GP presents herself as a doctor who complied with and supported the patient's need for narrative in her confused and desperate state. This, however, is immediately countered by the impact of clock time on the consultation and thus also on the storytelling situation: "but I said to her: 'Well, you know, we've cer——, I've [been] speaking for about twenty minutes. [I'm kind of] running out of time'" (line 11). The contrastive coordinator "but" clearly indicates a change in action (Schiffrin 1987), in this case the GP's interruption of the patient's narrative due to time constraints.

The fact that the GP repeats her words verbatim places an emphasis on this action and expresses the GP's feeling of pressure at the time. However, it also contradicts the GP's previously mentioned strategy of "going into that in detail." What remains to do in that situation, according to the doctor, is to initiate repeat visits: "So, get her to come back and some will come back, some won't. She did come back" (lines 12–14). The elliptical clause "some won't" indicates that lack of time can also keep patients away from the practice, but, as the GP contends almost apologetically in the final clause of the coda, "you do have to give them the chance to say it" (line 15). GPs' obligation to give patients opportunities to speak is emphasized by the auxiliary "do" and the modal "have to." Ironically, while the GP seems to be adamant about this facet of doctor-patient communication, her narrative illustrates important shortcomings of present-day medical practice exactly in that respect: narrative as a discursive genre is precluded in situations where patients may find this the only feasible means of communicating their problems.

Time, Self-Disclosure, and Narrative Production

Self-disclosure is generally seen as a "mechanism by which relationships become personal and intimate" (Brown and Rogers 1991:150). Applied to the particular case of disclosing domestic violence, this means that a certain degree of intimacy is established between patient and doctor or is even required prior to disclosure, which is incompatible with a rigid time frame. Where time is short, good psychological insight becomes necessary in general practice: "The ability to assess appropriately in a short space of time requires more than just listening skills; it requires a psychological understanding of the dynamics of presenting problems and what may underpin them" (Hudson-Allez 1997:6). As far as domestic violence victims are concerned, this understanding can best be achieved by narrative production (Lawless 2001). Narrative helps patients make sense of their lives not only for themselves but potentially also for their GP. Time pressure therefore obviously plays a significant role not only in making the consultation formal and impersonal but also in impeding greater psychological insight on the part of the GP. Time and the disclosure of domestic violence might be an even bigger issue for female doctors. The literature on self-disclosure (Brown and Rogers 1991:151–52) suggests that women in general (1) disclose more than men, (2) disclose about topics different from men's, (3) disclose more to other women than to men, and (4) receive disclosures from others more often than men do. Applied to women doctors, this means that they may be seen as more readily available for "emotional" talk, which in turn may put them under stronger pressure in a consultation.

Doctors' "Myth of Time"

In raising their lack of time as a central point during the interview the GPs evoked what Wodak calls doctors' "myth of time": "After all, the role cliché exists of the doctor who is constantly on call and thus permanently under pressure of time, and who corresponds to the 'prophylactic emergency behaviour'" (1997:194). Everyone seems to take it for a fact that GPs are very busy and that their time is more valuable than others'. As McKie, Fennell, and Mildorf demonstrate, responses such as "We are extremely busy," "We don't really have time," "There are so many calls on our time," "GPs' time is a premium" form "the starting point as well as the result of a dynamic, dialectic process in which GPs mythologise time, drawing upon various concepts and types of time, but at the same time reinforcing the time myth" (2002:332–33) in their narratives. Put another way, the time myth becomes an argument for a number of difficulties doctors may encounter in general practice, especially with regard to domestic violence cases and other "nonmedical" problems, and since the "fact" of lack of time is hardly challenged by doctors and patients alike, the argument always remains valid.

On the other hand, a consultation is undoubtedly limited by external time constraints imposed on general practice mainly because of financial considerations. The succinct "time is money" argument increasingly influences the health care system, and consequently the GPs' time is considered a resource that must be managed and accounted for. This puts the GP under pressure to keep the consultation within a set time frame. Consider the following comments, in which GPs discuss reasons why they would perhaps refrain from broaching the issue of domestic violence:

1. a. [I am] **reluctant only in terms of time constraints** during a particular consultation. I mean if, **if it's been going on for ages**, er, and I know that it would be a can of worms that would be opened, **I will maybe leave it.**

b. I mean I've seen women with clearly, er, [pause] domestic abuse injuries and they, they just don't say it, you know, and **sometimes you don't ask, depending on how long you, you have.**

c. And **I would never raise the subject in a ten minute consultation** un ——, unless the patient wants to.

d. Often people will come in with a very, um, minor complaint and they'll **woffle on about that for ages** and you say: "Right, well, is there anything else I can do for you?" 'cause you feel there probably is and then, you know, they burst into tears and say whatever and **that can be quite hard if that's sort of nine and a half minutes into your consultation** [laughs], I: "Oh, no!" but, you know, you still feel that you have to ask them.

e. Yeah, and then it's what, [sighs] what do you do thereafter, you know? Um, it shouldn't be an issue but partly the time issue as well. I mean **we've got seven and a half minutes, ten minutes and, um, it shouldn't be an issue but I think, in reality, it is.**

f. It is a **pressure type of consultation** for us, not so much for dealing with that individual but knowing that you've still got people who are waiting to see you inside as well.

g. We're not, um, **we don't have the time or resource[s] to deal with that.** We have **more and more illness** and, er, **more and more medi-**

cal things that we have to do. Our **workload is going up all the time** and this is a **time, er, consuming, er, subject** in the area.

Indeed, it can be easier for GPs within a limited consultation time not to open this "can of worms" (as the GP in [1a] put it, thereby drawing upon another metaphor I discussed in the previous chapter) than to face all the consequences and responsibilities a disclosure of domestic violence might trigger. Example (1d) exemplifies the situation where a patient simply needs more time to build up a narrative about her problem, and the doctor feels stressed by the length of this process ("Oh, no!"). On the other hand, doctors' feeling of constant time pressure may keep them from probing further even if they have a suspicion that domestic violence is at stake. This can be seen in the responses in (1a) and (1d), in which the GPs partly conjure up the "horror vision" of a patient suddenly opening up in a consultation "sort of nine and a half minutes into your consultation" (1d) and "if it's been going on for ages" (1a). Time is presented as an external factor GPs are not in control of.

Interestingly enough, however, the GPs were by and large also of the opinion that they could "make time" if that was necessary and that time constraints could always be circumvented by means of repeat visits, for example:

2. a. But the answer to the question "Do I have any hesitation in asking [about it]" is "no." **In case of timing, do I have to do it there and then, the answer to that question is also "no."** You don't have to dive in there and then, you say "Oh, there's a bruise," you say, "Er, **will you come back? I want to see you next week** and I want to give you a ten minute appointment or a double appointment." And then you say: "While you were in here last week I noticed that you had . . . "

b. Time is an issue and we have, we're on determined appointments from sort of two to fifteen minutes. So that gives a little leeway but, er, **we don't sit there with an egg timer** and **if there's a need for, to talk, we can let them go on to some extent.** And **if you run out of time** and there's obviously more to discuss then **they come back later.** There's also the facility for a long appointment at the end of the surgery if, if that's needed.

c. But I think, as a *GP*, you have to **allow one or two people extra time.**
And, um, I think it's one of the skills of the doctor to **work out who
needs it.** And I think you can always **ask people to come back.**

d. If it were a major problem, obviously you would just have to
make the time. You can't hurry them out in that situation. You've
got to accept that you're gonna be **delayed for another ten minutes**
while you try and, particularly if it's **the first time** you get to speaking about it, you can't really stop them and say: "Look, this isn't my
problem. Go to a social worker!" If you do that you're not gonna do
them any favors 'cause it might be the only, **the one and only time**
that they've spoken to somebody about it.

e. I mean, *GPs* always have this **excuse of lack of time** but, um, there's
no harm in running over the appointment time, you know, patients
don't mind waiting. They know that one day it might be them. Or
you can get the patient to come back. You can say: "Ah, it seems as
if we need to talk about it a bit more. Why don't you make an appointment or the last appointment in the surgery or a double appointment." It is possible.

Time becomes a double-edged sword in the GPs' discourse, which can be seen in
the way the GPs contradict themselves when they speak about their time management. On the one hand, time is presented as an external factor that the GPs
do not have control over and that therefore puts them under stress; on the other
hand, time is turned into an object that GPs can manipulate at will. So are GPs
in control of time or not? What are we supposed to make of the doctors' con-
tradictory representations of time? This is exactly where the idea of mythologizing comes into play. As Barthes contends: "Myth is a *value*, truth is no guarantee for it; nothing prevents it from being a perpetual alibi: it is enough that
its signifier has two sides for it always to have an 'elsewhere' at its disposal"
(1972:123, emphasis in original). The myth of time in a sense also becomes a
value during the interviews, a value that is constantly negotiated between the
GPs and the interviewer. To draw upon Bourdieu's (1991) metaphor of the linguistic marketplace, the topic of time becomes a discursive commodity that the
doctors in my sample tried to "sell" to the interviewer. Depending on the con-

text, time was attributed higher or lower "value." Thus, when doctors talked about general pressures involved in the treatment of domestic violence cases, time played a major role. As soon as they referred to themselves as professionals dealing with this issue, time lost its strength and was presented as flexible and possible to manipulate. The GP in (2e) even critically talks about the "excuse of lack of time," thus implying that the time myth is deliberately used by doctors to cover up other reasons for nonintervention. A problem arises when doctors internalize the time myth to such a degree that they become easily stressed by a disrupted schedule.

Doctors' myth of time can be even more harmful when the patients also internalize it. Women may feel that they should not make "unjustified" claims on their GP's time, or, as one GP put it, "people don't want to bother you if it's a waste of time." If we bear in mind that storytelling always requires both narrator and listener, since the listener tests ways of listening to and understanding the story (Hydén 1997), it becomes clear why patients sometimes feel that GPs are not accessible or receptive to their narratives. The time myth hinders doctors from spending more time with a patient, and patients do not feel they have the right to disturb the GP's tight schedule. Thus, GPs' mythologizing about time can ultimately influence their behavior toward patients in a consultation as well as the patients' behavior, and it is therefore not surprising that women who suffer abuse return to surgeries frequently before they finally manage to disclose. However, time was not the only argument put forth by the GPs to explain their rather passive role in domestic violence cases. In the following section I discuss the ways in which GPs conceptualized backgrounds of domestic abuse and hence defined their own professional role in domestic violence cases as inadequate.

Backgrounds and Explanations of Abuse

One of the questions I asked the GPs during the interviews was "Why do you think domestic violence happens at all?" or the similar question "What are the reasons for domestic violence?" This question elicited a wide range of responses that reveal GPs' concepts of and attitudes toward domestic abuse. Before I discuss these responses I would like to digress by presenting Ptacek's (1990) research on the way batterers explain their violent behavior. Following research conducted by Scott and Lyman (1968), Ptacek divides the explanations offered by the eighteen men he interviewed into two broad categories, *excuses* and *justifications*: "Excuses are those accounts in which the abuser denies full responsibility for his actions. Justifications are those accounts in which the batterer may accept some responsibility but denies or trivializes the wrongness of his violence" (1990:141). The denial of responsibility is mainly accomplished by an appeal to loss of control, on the one hand, and a strategy of victim blaming, on the other hand. Thus, batterers blamed the influence of alcohol or drugs for their behavior, or they described their violent attacks in terms of a frustration-aggression model, whereby the violence resulted from an accumulation of internal pressure. Violence was also reconstructed as a "response" to women's physical or verbal aggressiveness, which placed the blame for violence on the victim. One of the main strategies for denying that the violence was wrong is the trivialization of the women's injuries. Furthermore, batterers found fault with their partners, blaming their failure to fulfill the requirements of being a "good wife" such as cooking, willingness to have sex, deference, faithfulness, and so on. Ptacek argues that "these rationalizations represent culturally sanctioned strategies for minimizing and denying violence against women" (1990:151). In his article Ptacek examines the literature written by social workers, psychologists, psychiatrists, and other professionals directly involved in working with men who batter women:

> Most striking is that batterers and clinicians use similar language to characterize "loss of control." The batterers speak in terms of irrational attacks ("I went berserk"; "I wasn't sane"; "temporary insanity"); uncontrollable aggression ("I had no control over myself"; "it's a condition of being out of control"; "uncontrollably violent"); and explosion metaphors ("I just blew up"; "blowout"; "walking time bomb"; "outburst of rage"; "eruptions"). Like the batterers, many clinicians also describe the violence as irrational or psychopathological. (1990:152)

In a similar vein Ptacek argues that clinicians accept batterers' rationalizations for the violence with regard to victim blaming. The conclusion Ptacek puts forward at the end is that the excuses and justifications he outlines in his study are "ideological constructs": "At the individual level, they obscure the batterers' self-interest in acting violently; at the societal level, they mask the male domination underlying violence against women. Clinical and criminal justice responses to

battering are revealed as ideological in the light of their collusion with batterers' rationalizations" (1990:155). In other words, discourses help (re)construct
and perpetuate conceptualizations of domestic violence that are based on myths
and informed by patriarchal ideologies. Since I subscribe to the same view, I investigated the GPs' responses in my sample with a view to identifying excuses
and justifications for violent behavior.

If we extract explanations out of all the interviews, it is possible to list a seemingly wide range of reasons. Responses included the following twelve broad
factors:

1. Alcohol or drug abuse
2. Deprivation and low social background
3. Family history of violence and socialization process
4. Lack of education
5. Lack of communication and social skills and conflict resolution
   by means of physical force
6. Relationship problems
7. Aggression and jealousy
8. Biological preconditions such as physical size and power
9. Male dominance and viewing the partner as property
10. Men's feeling of inadequacy and threat through women's grow-
    ing independence
11. Manifestation of affection
12. Women's low status in some cultures

Many of these explanations can be mapped onto Ptacek's out-of-control or
blame-the-victim strategies. Thus, for example, the reasons in 1 through 4 locate the problem outside the perpetrator's power, that is, violence is said to happen because of external factors rather than because the man wants it to happen.
Relationship problems and jealousy are problematic as explanations, since they
suggest that part of the problem is also the woman's fault. Although all these
items, taken together, convey a picture of variation and balance in the GPs' responses, we must not forget that some of these explanations were offered by
only a few doctors and thus do not necessarily represent mainstream lines of
reasoning. Thus, only a few female GPs alluded to the reason given in 9, namely,
that domestic abuse can be interpreted as a result of men's dominant status in

society and some men's tendency to view women as property, while the explanations offered in 10 and 11 primarily occurred in explicit terms in some of the male GPs' responses. All the doctors in my sample provided a mixture of some of the reasons above, and by far the commonest explanations across all the interviews, regardless of age or gender of the GP, were the ones stated in 1 to 5. It is important to note that these are mostly explanations that researchers on domestic violence have identified as common cultural myths as outlined in chapter 3. In a sense, by drawing upon these explanations GPs indirectly reinforce and perpetuate already existing myths that stigmatize victims and thus also contribute to a further tabooing of the issue.

Stereotypical Scenarios: Alcohol, Low Social Background, and a Family History of Abuse

Doctors also contradicted themselves, for example, when they stated that the problem of domestic violence was multifactorial but then went on to linguistically present scenarios of social deprivation, alcohol-related violence, and drug abuse. The following responses illustrate this point:

> 3. a. I don't think we were ever taught anything about it. Er, we were told that it existed, that it was a **social phenomenon,** you know, part of the **Saturday night ritual of husband getting plastered after the football match, going home and beating up his wife, and falling asleep.** The sort of thing that we regularly saw when I was working in casualty in the late sixties but we never really thought it was, er, a, as **widespread** and as **malignant** a problem as I think it's probably turned out to be.

> b. There might be somebody who **goes out and gets pissed and [lives in a] horrible neighborhood** and, so that's all distressing, they're **unemployed and all that sort of stuff, then beats up his wife.** It's not a health issue.

> c. You know, I mean, sometimes there is a **background of, of drug taking,** er, often **alcohol use,** both by one or both partners, er, I think **sometimes people are difficult to live with and people find difficulty living with each other** and, and depending on er, er, **their own**

parenting, the way that they'd been brought up and their expectations of what living in a partnership is about, er, and, er, whether they have discovered that, er, life is about sharing and not being selfish or, I mean just, I mean learning how to live. Um, many of them **don't have those skills** and I think when they find themselves in, er, a close relationship, I mean close physically in, you're living, you know, in the same space, er, with different ideas about, er, what to do with the money that's coming into the household or how to bring up the children or **what drugs to take that night or, you know, let's go out and get smashed on a Friday night,** you know, [?]. Um, they find it difficult to cope.

Interestingly enough, these scenarios were conjured up by male GPs, while female doctors were less likely to dramatize their explanations of domestic abuse, although they also mentioned alcohol and drugs as frequent triggers of violence. The GPs create what they perceive as typical scenes of domestic abuse and even accommodate their speech in terms of colloquialisms and lower register in order to mimic the kind of language a batterer might use: "getting plastered," "gets pissed," and "get smashed." The scenarios are also interesting because they draw upon stereotypical notions of what men usually do: they go out on a Friday night or watch a football match on Saturday, get drunk, and then beat up their partners. The GP in (3a) sees domestic violence as part of a "ritual" that has turned out to be far more "malignant" and "widespread." In other words, as long as domestic violence can be explained as part of this Saturday night ritual in connection with alcohol it can be understood and dealt with, whereas nowadays it seems to be far more subtle and deviant. Ironically, the GP depicts domestic violence in medical terms, as one would talk about ulcers or carcinoma, although he states that domestic violence is a "social phenomenon."

Example (3b) illustrates the correlation that GPs draw between social factors and abuse. The logical and temporal connector "then" links up domestic violence in a causal relationship with unemployment and poor housing conditions, which are emphasized in the judgmental expanded noun phrase "horrible neighborhood." In (3c) the GP provides a lengthy explanation with numerous factors, but all these explanations are linguistically embedded in a framework of notions of drug taking and alcohol abuse. Thus, the GP starts his explanation by mentioning exactly those two factors, and he ends by almost cynically enacting the way such drug taking or alcoholism might manifest itself in a relationship. Another middle-aged male GP mentioned power dynamics within relationships and the potential threat some men may perceive, but he then almost ridicules the whole argument by conjuring up a scene where a batterer plans his violent behavior, again in connection with alcohol and against the background of the going-out ritual:

> 4. [One could have] some sociological theory, I mean, power in a relationship and the [other] dynamic within a relationship, er, and the use of power in a relationship. Or the abuse of power. . . . And, it happens when there's a threat, or one party sees a threat to their position within a relationship for whatever reason [?] in terms of their freedom that "I want to **go out with the boys and get pissed** and I come back and then, you know, you're going to be my slave and you [do what I want you to do]."

The most striking feature in this scenario is the use of "constructed dialogue" (Tannen 1989:110). Constructed dialogue, which is marked by the insertion of direct speech in an account or a narrative, is often used in conversation because it "creates involvement by both its rhythmic, sonorous effect and its internally evaluative effect" (Tannen 1989:133). Here it is supposed to convey the batterer's thoughts or even words with which he addresses his wife, and it is mainly used to give life to the scene. By drawing upon such a cliché this GP trivializes the problem and neglects wider issues concerning male dominance that pervade our society. As the literature on domestic violence demonstrates, violence can be triggered but not ultimately caused by alcohol abuse. Johnson (2001), for example, contends that men do not batter their partners because they are intoxicated but because they have the power to do it (see chapter 3). In contrast to example (4), consider the following comment made by an older female GP who discusses the same issue and also uses constructed direct speech:

> 5. I don't think men identify that actually overtly. Um, **I think it's just something they do.** They don't sort of think, "Right," I m——, I mean, I don't think they think consciously "Right, I'm the one to take that power over you," um, it just happens.

This GP presents the question of power in much more universal terms. That men exert power over women is "just something they do" and is thus regarded as a mechanism ingrained in society as a whole. Nevertheless, most of the responses reveal that explanations such as alcohol are often used by doctors as excuses not necessarily to condone but to understand violent acts. As I said above, such explanations are problematic in that they divert attention from more fundamental questions concerning power and the acceptance of violence in our society. These explanations have such a strong standing in general social discourses that even victims themselves absorb and reproduce them, as one young female GP pointed out: "I think some women accept it because their hus ——, their husband only does it when he's drunk, because they believe it's the drink talking rather than the, the chap talking." The personification of "the drink" points toward a strategy GPs also regularly adopt in their explanations, namely, to assign agentive power to social problems of all sorts and thus to deflect the issue away from the male perpetrator.

Even where the perpetrator was moved into focus, which only occurred when GPs were specifically asked about reasons for domestic abuse, the violence was mostly explained in terms of external factors. In the following response a middle-aged female GP rationalizes batterers' behavior by drawing upon the typical family history explanation mentioned above and in chapter 3 as well as on personal character, but the personality explanation is then supplemented by a kind of biological excuse that men are physically stronger than women and therefore resort to violence:

> 6. And some of it is because **that's what they've seen as children** as well so that **it's not unusual to hit mum** if you're, if **you come home and you're annoyed** or you maybe have seen that and, and that can, that can lead them but, um, I mean I know it, it does happen in more affluent areas as well. It's unfair to say it's all because of deprivation but, I mean, I think a lot of it must be personality in the person that does it and then they **need to be in control** and, and **the only way** possibly in the relationship they can do that is **physically usually** 'cause the **man is more powerful than the woman.**

The scenario of the family violence background is conjured up through the use of the colloquial noun "mum" and the generic pronoun "you," which creates a sense of general applicability. The shift from "they" to generic "you" also indicates a shift from the speaker's distant position closer to the point of view of the "children" because "you" indirectly also includes the speaker. Thus, the GP indicates that she can understand how these things come about, or, in her own words, "you can see how it can happen." The GP then moves on to an explanation based on the perpetrator's personality. Batterers "need to be in control," and the "only way" to achieve this is by physical violence, because "the man is more powerful than the woman." By using the attributive adjective "only" and by applying generics for "man" and "woman," the GP makes quite a categorical statement about the correlation between a sense of power, physical strength, and violence, thereby reconstructing another common cliché. The biological fact that men are physically stronger is thus used to locate violent behavior within a feasible explanatory framework.

The Construction and Reiteration of Cognitive Maps and Explanatory Frameworks

By conjuring up specific backgrounds against which domestic violence occurs, doctors also create cognitive maps yet on a more abstract, conceptual level. The various backgrounds of deprived lives, poverty, underachievement, drug taking, alcohol abuse, family violence, and so on function as cognitive frameworks within which domestic violence can be comfortably located, identified, and understood. In terms of theories of narrative knowledge (see chapter 2), the GPs (re-)create specific narratives about possible causes of domestic violence in order to categorize and compartmentalize the problem and to make it thus comprehensible. In other words, my analyses show narrative to function as an ordering principle for people's "transactions," in this case, GPs' rationalizations of a problem they encounter in their practice work. If the setting of violence does not conform to the general or schematized cognitive map of violence, doctors express their surprise or find the violence incomprehensible. Thus, one GP commented that "it's often been surprising to me, er, people I've known for a long, long time, who've seemed like very decent, er, people, very, er, decent families, decent relationships, suddenly came out with domestic violence problems." In other words, domestic abuse is more unexpected in "decent" people, that is, presumably, people from a standard middle-class background, than in people from a background GPs are maybe less familiar with as far as their own personal experience is concerned. Another older male GP related a narrative of one of his patients and concluded by saying "and she was a, you know, nice, decent person." Again, the attribute of being decent is depicted as a contrast to people's involvement in domestic abuse. The implication is that it is incomprehensible that a nice person could be subjected to violence or, put differently, that she could have done anything to deserve violence. Thus, the doctor established an implicit link between the occurrence of violence and the victim's behavior that corresponds with the victim-blaming strategy mentioned above.

Doctors' cognitive maps of domestic violence also locate abuse in a socially remote place. Most GPs acknowledged that, statistically speaking, domestic abuse occurs across all social classes and in all areas. Nevertheless, GPs' scenarios and narratives in the interviews depict predominantly deprived social backgrounds. This indicates that doctors cognitively map abuse onto spatial regions that they themselves do not inhabit, and thus they once again create a distance or at least some kind of "comfort zone" between themselves and their patients. We may object here that detachment is part of GPs' job and that they are trained to keep their distance and not become too emotionally involved. This standpoint is problematic, however, if it leads to GPs' early resignation in view of domestic violence cases or, even worse, to their deliberate neglect of the issue. By drawing upon the common excuses and justifications outlined by Ptacek (1990), GPs reinforce cultural myths and stereotypes about domestic abuse and, at the same time, widen the gap between patients and the medical profession. Thus, miscommunication and misconceptions that lead to mutual dissatisfaction and frustration are likely to persist in general practice and therefore perpetuate a need for special training, as Williamson contends:

> As with all of these explanations, it is important to consider the wider social and political framework within which domestic violence occurs. This includes acknowledging the historical and cultural acceptance of violence against women on a global scale. That such theories were relatively common in the interviews with stage two participants suggests that much more work needs to be conducted in challenging social myths and stereotypes about domestic violence, in the context of general basic awareness training. (2000:99)

In the final chapter I return to the issue of training and especially address the need for a training module on narrative communication in medicine.

In addition, the explanations mentioned above define domestic violence predominantly within the social rather than the medical realm and thus keep the problem out of doctors' sphere of activities and responsibilities. In the following sections I address the question of doctors' agency.

The Discursive Construction of "Medical" and "Social" Problems

GPs did not see their role as being "experts" in domestic violence; instead, they emphasized their function as "generalists" or as "general practice specialists" who were "just expected to do too many things" and therefore did not regard it as their task to prioritize domestic violence. As one male GP put it: "I don't want to be a specialist in domestic violence." This phrase is meaningful, as it reveals GPs' defensiveness about their work and position within the medical setting. Unlike doctors who specialize in a particular field, GPs are expected to know a lot about many different things. However, their rank in the hierarchy of doctors is considerably lower and their job less appreciated than that of other types of doctors. As Annandale points out, "GPs have historically enjoyed less power and status than senior hospital doctors, although their relative isolation has tended to afford them a fairly high degree of clinical autonomy" (1998:241). Statements such as the ones above may indicate GPs' dissatisfaction with their lower status. However, the GPs thus also separated "medical" from "social" problems, and they indirectly set up limitations to their own responsibilities. The following narrative illustrates this point. It was related by an older female doctor in the context of a discussion of the status of domestic violence in the health care setting. The narrative refers to an incident that occurred while the GP was on duty with the regional emergency doctors (G-Docs = Grampian Doctors).

Narrative 9

1. I was in G-Docs, er, just a few weeks ago,
2. and, er, I was called out to something with, you know, that was a domestic violence situation.
3. Um, it was kind of given a lower status than or a low——, lower priority than say, maybe an elderly person with a stroke or a heart attack or something like that.
4. So, you know, it was kind of a nuisance that we had to go out and see it

5. and, er, then they got the social workers involved
6. and I say I think they kind of think, "Well, it's the social workers' problem, it's not ours," you know,
7. and the police were involved as well, so,
8. they left it with the social workers, so.
9. Poor social workers, that's not fair [laughs].

In this narrative the GP openly, albeit tentatively, addresses the problem that domestic violence is often given low priority by doctors. The hedge "kind of" in lines 3, 4, and 6 ("kind of given lower status," "kind of a nuisance," "they kind of think") indicates that the GP implicitly wishes to downplay the fact that domestic violence was not taken too seriously by the doctors and thus to maintain her "face wants" (Goffman 1967), namely, not to be viewed critically herself by the interviewer. Higher up on GPs' agenda and thus presumably also at the forefront of their attention, as the GP hypothesizes by using the modal adverbial "maybe" in line 3 ("maybe an elderly person with a stroke"), we can find a disease such as a "stroke" or a "heart attack" (line 3) that is easily identifiable as a prototypical "medical" problem. Interestingly enough, the GP compartmentalizes such diseases by placing them in the same category, as can be seen in the extended noun phrase "something like that" (line 3). Although the category remains unspecified, the GP nonetheless indirectly draws a distinctive line between "medical" and "other" problems.

In the case of domestic violence the emergency doctors find it "a nuisance" to "go out and see it" (line 4). The postposition "out" in "called out" (line 2) and "go out" (line 4) evokes both the container metaphor and the path schema whereby the doctors are forced to leave their secluded medical sphere ("*in* G-Docs," my emphasis), especially as the roles are reversed in this particular setting and the doctors now assume the part of the "moving actor" who approaches the patient. This spatiotemporal condition combined with the above-mentioned partition between "medical" and "other" problems discursively creates a seemingly valid reason for doctors' discontent. In other words, since domestic violence is not a medical problem, it does not justify that they are called out. Consequently, the GP expresses her own irritation in that situation, and she establishes a division of duties for doctors and social workers in the direct quotation of her colleagues' alleged thoughts: "Well, it's the social workers' problem, it's not ours" (line 6). The quote has as its central theme the delegation of further responsibility to other agencies, and the fact that the GP uses the alleged thoughts of others to express this view also reveals the mechanisms of "face work" (Goffman 1967) and "interpersonal perception" (Laing, Phillipson, and Lee 1966). In order to avoid potential criticism on the part of the interviewer and to save her own face, the GP "hides" her own opinion behind the one of her colleagues. The shift from the deictic center "I" (line 2: "I was called out") to "we" (line 4: "we had to go out") to "they" (lines 5, 6, and 8: "they got the social workers involved," "they kind of think," "they left it") and the use of passive constructions, which usually blur agency (Jackendoff 2002:248), in lines 3 and 7 ("it was kind of given a lower status," "the police were involved") contribute to a certain discursive "self-defense." At the same time, however, the narrative itself reinforces on a microlinguistic level exactly those concepts that the GP seems to acknowledge as being problematic or at least open to criticism on the surface. Thus, for example, the delegation of responsibility to other "social actors" is captured by the contrast between the frequently and fully spelled out noun phrase "social workers" in lines 5, 6, 8, and 9 and the replacement of the noun phrase "G-Docs" by its reduced form, the personal pronoun "they," in lines 5, 6, and 8. In a sense, the social workers are thus granted fuller cognitive presence in the narrative and, hence, more importance, while the GPs appear only as marginal actors in this situation. Likewise, the domestic violence case as such is marginalized in the narrative by means of underspecification through the vague pronoun "something" and the indefinite determiner "a" in line 2 ("a domestic violence situation") as well as its further linguistic reduction through the pronoun "it" (lines 3, 4, 6, and 8). These rather tentative descriptors indicate the GP's reluctance to label the incidence in terms of domestic violence and perhaps also her embarrassment at speaking about the issue.

Despite the GP's awareness that doctors' refusal to prioritize domestic violence can be problematic, the narrative undermines this message by linguistically replicating the same refusal. It also demonstrates how deeply the GP's discourse is immersed in and informed by the biomedical model, which justifies the low priority of domestic violence on GPs' agenda because it leads doctors away from the clearly demarcated "pathway" prescribed by mainstream medicine and thrusts on them a responsibility that they do not perceive as part of their social role as medical professionals. As I mentioned in the previous chapter, one young female GP used the metaphor of the "medical wardrobe" in which domestic abuse does not fit; she continued: "So, as you can't treat it, um, you know, we don't have a very big role to play in that." In other words, if there is nothing physically wrong with a patient, the GP cannot do much. Consider also the following responses:

7. a. There's **nae very much I can really do** about domestic violence.

b. I think giving them sympathy but **that's about it.**

c. It's difficult 'cause it's not, **there's not like a cure for it.**

d. I kind of think: "Oh, heaven's sakes, **what am I going to do here?**" because it's not really something you can, you can help people with in a kind of "sorting it" way, you know, you can help and support them but **you can't really fix it for them.**

e. You feel a bit **powerless** actually. There's **not an awful lot you can do** for them.

f. You **can't really necessarily change the situation for them,** you know.

g. **I don't feel there's an awful lot practical we can do** to support them. It's usually referring on to other agencies.

h. **Social services may be better placed** to deal with this type of thing.

i. [It is] [s]omething I'm **ill equipped to deal with.**

Again, the answers are strikingly similar, and this is only a small selection of responses, all of which follow the same linguistic pattern: negators combined with the quantifiers "much" and "a lot," which are sometimes strengthened by the intensifiers "very" or "awful." In (7c), (7d), and (7g) the presuppositions of the medical framework shine through, assigning doctors the power to deal with a physical problem "practically" by means of "fixing it" with "cures." In the case of psychosocial symptoms, however, GPs are "ill equipped" and feel "power-less." By frequently evoking these adjectives in their narratives the GPs created another myth, namely, the myth of their own inadequacy when faced with do-mestic violence cases. This myth, if generally accepted as a fact, may well hin-der GPs from adopting a more active role.

It is not surprising that the vocabulary most of the GPs used when they spoke about their role also conveyed a sense of the "clinical" approach to domestic violence:

> 8. a. Well, if she's got **signs** of physical abuse I would **examine her** and find out if she's got any injuries, the **nature of the injuries,** the **extent of the injuries.**

> b. So, often at a first disclosure, it's only appropriate to **note it,** to ask a little bit more about the circumstances, what's happening **in terms of physical stuff.**

> c. Yes, my role is mainly, I suppose, **medical or supportive.**

> d. And in that situation obviously, um, we listen, we **record** what happened, we **record any injuries.**

> e. I think as GPs, our job is to try and **identify it,** um, and try to help as much as we can but I think ultimately, I think it's an ongoing problem we end up referring onward to the others.

> f. I think for the GP the main job is to **detect the problem** and find out, is there a readiness to do something about it? And if there is, facilitate the first steps and involve whoever needs to be involved to do something.

> g. Most of the women have come to **have injuries cataloged.**

> h. What can you do? What are the **immediate needs?** You know, is there **anything broken,** is there anything that needs some sort of **treatment?**

i. We're not mind readers and if we're having a busy surgery and, all we see is the **pink page in front of us.** We're not looking through notes all the time and analyze everybody's consultation. So **if they come in with a sore throat we deal with their sore throat** and then they go.

j. And then you know, depending on what they want to do, we would see them as regularly after that even if it's just as **support capacity** or **treating a depression.**

k. I have **documented the intrusion** and I have said to her I'd be willing to support her.

The responses illustrate to what extent the GPs' narratives are informed by scientific and bureaucratic discourses surrounding medical practice. Thus, domestic violence has to be "identified" (8e) and "detected" (8f) through physical "signs" (8a) just like other diseases caused by natural aggressors such as bacteria or viruses, and a normal institutional procedure is to "examine" (8a) the patient and to "document" (8k), "record" (8d), or "catalog" (8g) any physical injuries. The patient is thus implicitly reduced to the "pink page" (8i; see also chapter 5) in front of the doctor; that is, the "deciphering gaze" (Young 1995) is more or less restricted to the signs and symptoms that have entered the medical record and thus medical discourse on the patient's case history. By drawing upon biomedical discourse, GPs in a way also create a "comfort zone" for themselves, as they can use nonemotional language, which furthermore signals their membership in a specific professional group. Couser observes for medical jargon that "the opacity and impersonality of this language may provide necessary distance for the patient as well as the doctor, though its purpose is apparently to ease the physician's, rather than the patient's, suffering" (1997:26). Undoubtedly, to deal with cases of domestic violence can be emotionally taxing. A problem arises when doctors' emotions become so overpowering that they impede action.

Myths of Powerlessness and Inadequacy

The theme of powerlessness runs predominantly through the female GPs' responses, whereas male GPs seem to be more likely to reconstruct the medical/social divide in their discourses in order to justify their lack of response and action. Both explanations can be considered myths to the extent that they do not necessarily represent what is "true" but what medical doctors "believe to be true." As I argued in chapter 3, general practice is in fact well placed to discover and to subsequently deal with domestic violence. However, GPs' sense of being inadequately prepared in situations in which they encounter domestic violence in patients was sometimes so strong during the interview that the GPs incorporated it into their narratives or even made it the main focus of a story. In Labov's (1972a) terminology inadequacy as a theme is given enough importance to become "reportable." The following story related by a young female GP from a practice bordering on the city center illustrates this mechanism:

Narrative 34

1. I had, er, a girl who,
2. oh, it was so strange,
3. who was, she, the story was she'd fallen down the stairs and at the bottom of the stairs there was a glass door.
4. She'd fallen down the stairs and through the door
5. and her leg was in ribbons
6. and I sat about an hour stitching it up,
7. and her husband was a drug [user]
8. and he sat with me, the whole hour, saying sweet things in her ear, you know, and, you know, being generally supportive and ^so nice and ^so kind.
9. And then when she came back to the dressing clinic, to st——, to have her stitches out and see how her leg was doing,
10. she admitted that he'd actually pushed her through a glass door and that he'd been violent towards her for a long time.
11. But he wasn't, you know, he obviously wasn't there, um, at that point.
12. So, that was great she told me
13. and that gave me great in——, insight into what's been happening
14. but I felt then totally unprepared to do anything about it.
15. I mean I did nothing.

   16. I did nothing.

   17. I sympathized with her,

   18. I sent her on her way because, you know, we hadn't been told,

   19. I mean there's the A&E [accident and emergency] training

   20. but nobody ever mentioned issues of domestic violence.

   21. Perhaps they do now, that was, um, ten years ago.

The narrative starts with a clause typical of most of the narratives in my sample. It introduces the protagonist in a complex noun phrase, "a girl who was." The expansion of the noun phrase is interrupted, however, by the insertion of a clause that already gives a first evaluative statement before the story is actually told: "oh, it was so strange." The discourse marker "oh" is very interesting as it indicates the shift in information management at this point. As Schiffrin contends, "*oh* pulls from the flow of information in discourse a temporary focus of attention which is the target of self and/or other management" (1987:74). In this case, attention is drawn away from the actual storyline to the speaker's feelings about the story.

In the complicating action sequence two more actors appear on the scene: the doctor, who "sat about an hour stitching" up the patient's leg, and the patient's husband, who is immediately characterized in negative tones by the GP's mention of his drug addiction. The narrative action is situated temporally by the explicit reference to the duration of the treatment, "one hour," which is underlined by the use of the progressive form in "stitching" (line 6) and "saying" (line 8). The progressive form indicates the speaker's perception of this time period as long, and it might hint at a certain degree of discomfort felt by the GP in that situation. Another interesting linguistic feature in line 8 is the almost immediate repetition of the discourse marker "you know," which is used to create involvement: "and he sat with me, the whole hour, saying sweet things in her ear, you know, and, you know, being generally supportive." Obviously, the narrator reaches a point in her story where she becomes more emotional, and this is conveyed linguistically to the listener.

The resolution of the story, however, is suspended until line 10, where the truth is finally revealed. It comes out that, underlying the whole narrative, there is a history of domestic abuse. After the narrative proper the narrator adds a lengthy coda that gives room for the retrospective evaluation of the story. The evaluation section at the end is considerably longer than one would normally expect. This indicates that the point elaborated in this part is of major importance to the narrator. What is interesting here is that this narrative, like the narrative at the outset of the book and other narratives in my sample, lacks narrative closure in the sense that the woman's story remains unfinished.

Inactivity and a Feeling of Powerlessness as "Reportable Events" in Narrative 34

The coda from lines 12 to 21 summarizes what the GP thinks in retrospect about the whole story: "So, that was great she told me." The discourse marker "so" clearly demarcates the end of the preceding narrative and indicates to the listener that something else is to follow. In lines 12 and 13 the incident is evaluated positively as an experience that gave the GP "great insight": "So, that was great she told me and that gave me great in——, insight into what's been happening." The positive side is emphasized through the repetition of the adjective "great" in this context. However, this is soon countered with the contrastive coordinator "but," which introduces a negative facet of the GP's experience, namely, the fact that she was "unprepared to do anything." This is intensified by the adverb "totally." In line 15 the speaker marks, by using "I mean," her attention to the meaning of the statement she made in line 14 ("but I felt then totally unprepared to do anything"): "I mean I did nothing." The meaning of the sentence in line 14 is further clarified to the listener, and the GP quite literally "makes herself plain" by using a simple main clause to express her inaction: "I did nothing." The GP's sense of being almost paralyzed by her patient's story is reenacted by the structure of this narrative, where the coda brings everything to an uncommonly long halt. The coda furthermore reveals the *socionarrative* nature of the story, as it is mainly marked by discourse markers used to enhance speaker participation and mutual understanding. "You know" in line 18, for example, is used by the GP to make sure that the interviewer understands why it was so difficult for her to act appropriately in that situation: "I sent her on her way because, you know, we hadn't been told." In lines 17 to 20 the GP explains her reaction and her lack of agency through lack of training ("I sent her on her way because, you know, we hadn't been told, I mean there's the A&E training but nobody ever mentioned issues of domestic violence").

Voicing a Lack of Agency and Self-Criticism

At the end of the story the GP focuses on her own lack of action and thus presents herself as an unintentional agent of the woman's victimization: she actively "sends her on her way." This particular story as part of the GP's "storied knowledge" (Polkinghorne 1995) about domestic violence is retrieved at this stage of the interview in order to illustrate a point, namely, that there is a lack of appropriate training for GPs as far as domestic violence is concerned. The length of the coda shows that the evaluation of this story is important, since it focuses on the GP's experience of inadequacy rather than on the incident related in the story as such. This also suggests that this experience must have had a great psychological impact on the doctor. The GP by telling this story almost makes an apologetic gesture here. At another point in the interview the same GP criticizes herself openly when she says:

> 9. But I'm maybe very bad, I don't actually fit, pick up the phone
> and phone Grampian Women's Aid and make an appointment or
> write a letter. I, I basically I usually put it back to the girl to contact
> them and I don't know if that's, I mean how many of them actually
> do contact them or not I'm not sure.

This self-criticism hints at the mechanisms of interpersonal perception underlying the interview situation. By criticizing herself and by placing this self-criticism in an adequate explanatory frame (e.g., lack of training, insufficient experience, etc.) this GP linguistically anticipates potential criticism on the part of the interviewer and thus presents herself in a more favorable light as a GP who is self-conscious and aware of problematic issues surrounding her work with regard to domestic violence.

Summary

In this chapter I considered a number of myths the GPs drew upon and (re-)created in their narratives. On the one hand, the GPs' explanations of domestic violence were shown to be influenced by common cultural myths surrounding the problem, for example, the myths of causal relationships between social deprivation and violence or between alcohol abuse and violence. On the other hand,

I also demonstrated to what extent such explanations are used by GPs to delegate responsibility to society at large as domestic violence is reframed as a social rather than a medical problem. Another myth, the "myth of time" in general practice, proved to be another powerful discursive device to explain and to excuse doctors' reluctance to tackle domestic violence more actively. The question of agency is a crucial one when considering domestic violence and the health care system. For this reason I devote the following chapter to the investigation of the GPs' conceptualizations of the women's as well as their own agency.

7. Agents of Their Own Victimization
The Women's Role in the GPS' Narratives

"Why do they stay?" is a question commonly asked by GPS when they try to rationalize the behavior of patients who suffer domestic violence, and it is also a question almost all the GPS in my sample asked and answered at some point during the interview. However, this question becomes problematic if the GPS' explanations convey a picture of the woman as incompetent (Loseke and Cahill 1984). What is also at stake here is a question of agency, which can be viewed from two perspectives: the woman's relationship with her abusive partner, on the one hand, and the GP's role as provider of salient help, on the other. The analytic parts in this chapter therefore have the following twofold structure. First, I illustrate how female victims of domestic violence are linguistically presented and how GPS construct specific images of and identities for their patients. Second, this is complemented by an analysis of the way GPS conceptualize their own role as health care providers, which I partially also explored in the previous chapter. Here I investigate how general practitioners linguistically encode their role vis-à-vis the victims' behavior in their narratives. The analysis focuses in particular on the way passive constructions and modalities in the doctors' narratives set up and, at the same time, reinforce conceptual and expectational frames as well as evaluative parameters by which doctors judge their patients.

Modalities, for example, may reveal doctors' attitudes toward the factuality and significance of cases and thus also their expectations concerning women's behavior and lifestyle. According to Quirk et al.'s *Comprehensive Grammar of the English Language*, "*modality* may be defined as the manner in which the meaning of a clause is qualified so as to reflect the speaker's judgment of the likelihood of the proposition it expresses being true" (1985:219). One can distinguish between *intrinsic modality* such as "permission," "obligation," and "volition," which involve some kind of intrinsic human control over events, and *extrinsic modality* such as "possibility," "necessity," and "prediction," which do not primarily involve human control of events but do typically involve human judgment of what is or is not likely to happen. Leech's (1987) tripartite division of the notion of likelihood into *factual, theoretical,* and *hypothetical* meaning is also useful here. Factual meaning implies that the speaker takes the proposition for a fact, whereas theoretical meaning states a proposition as an idea rather than as fact. In Leech's terminology a factual sentence can be said to be "truth-committed," while a theoretical sentence is "truth-neutral" (1987:114). Hypothetical sentences, by contrast, imply the speaker's assumption that "the happening described did not, does not, or will not take place" (Leech 1987:118). Leech calls this condition "negative truth-commitment." Modal verbs also express factual, theoretical, or hypothetical meaning.

As modals indicate the speaker's judgment of the likelihood of an event, this could yield interesting results in the GPs' narratives about their patients. Thus, doctors might not consider a patient's presentation of domestic abuse in the home credible or likely, or they might create a scenario of a relationship using the indicative mood without even knowing what the real situation is. When GPs talk about consultations with patients, they might frequently use modals such as "would" or "could," thereby implying that the whole depiction is more a theoretical or even hypothetical construct than an account based on real-life experience. At the same time, modals expressing obligation might reveal how GPs judge and evaluate the victim's role in terms of agency, for example. Modals can also be used as a means of verbal distancing from a situation and may thus indicate the GPs' lack of understanding or involvement. Some of these possibilities are explored in the narratives presented in this chapter.

Moreover, in order to illustrate how "agency" in particular is constructed in the GPs' discourses and used as a "commodity" in the sense of Bourdieu's (1991) "linguistic market place," I draw in this chapter mainly on linguistic theta theory, with its thematic roles of *agens* and *patiens* (Gruber 1965; Fillmore 1968; Jackendoff 1972) and Goffman's (1974) frame theory as well as the sociopsychological concept of role negotiation. After all, as Bruner (1986) argues, meaning and human cognition only manifest themselves in people's discussions and negotiations of concepts (see chapter 2).

Actors and Agents

Before I proceed with the analysis, the terms *actors* and *agents*, which I introduce in the title of this section, require some clarification. The term *actor* is borrowed from Goffman's (1974) frame theory. As I briefly outlined in chapter 3, Goffman conceptualized conversation as a staged play during which participants act out their roles as individuals but also as social and professional personae. The concept of "frame" includes organizational rules for interaction on both a social as well as a personal level. Thus, Goffman assumes that "definitions of a situation are built up in accordance with principles of organization which govern events—at least social ones—and our subjective involvement in them" (1974:10–11). Goffman distinguishes between "natural" and "social" frameworks, and the main difference between these two is the way individuals are conceptualized with regard to agency:

> A central difference between natural and social frameworks is the
> role accorded actors, specifically individuals. In the case of natu
> ral perspectives, individuals have no special status, being subject
> to the same deterministic, will-less, nonmoral way of being as any
> other part of the scene. In the case of social frameworks, individ
> uals figure differently. They are defined as self-determined agen
> cies, legally competent to act and morally responsible for doing so
> properly. In this latter connection, then, individuals have an en
> tirely special role in activity. Moreover, this role is diffusely rele
> vant. The properties we attribute to normal actors, such as correct
> perception, personal will, a range of adult competencies, access
> to memory, a measure of empathy regarding others present, hon
> esty, reliability, fixed social and personal identity, and the like are
> counted on in a multitude of ways whenever interpersonal deal
> ings occur. (1974:188)

The notion of social frames and of participants' expectations underlying interaction can also be transferred onto the consultation, during which doctor and patient are the actors in a more or less predetermined sequence of events: presentation, examination, and diagnosis of illness, as well as the initiation of treatment and remedy. In chapters 2 and 5 I mentioned Strong (1979), who refers to the almost ritual procedures in medical encounters as the "ceremonial order," that is, the fact that both doctor and patient act out their expected roles in the consultation frame and that they try to reach an agreeable conclusion to their conversation. Young observes that framing in medical examinations "is accomplished by greetings, forms of address, language about the body, deference and dominance behavior, costuming, role play, the management of verbal and nonverbal delicacy, ritual, and metacommunication" (1997:11). The transactional nature of medical encounters, as in any other socially organized service encounter,[1] requires that participants' expectations of the interaction are met; otherwise, they can lead to misunderstandings and disappointment.

In consultations where domestic violence is at stake, the GP might, for example, expect to follow the biomedical consultation model with presentation, examination, and diagnosis, while the patient hopes to gradually open up about her problem, possibly assisted by appropriate prompts offered by the doctor (see chapter 5). Very often, doctors' discursive practices are influenced, for example, by the requirements of record keeping, as Ainsworth-Vaughn points out: "First, physicians often have certain specific goals that they must accomplish during the talk. They have (justifiably) been required to memorize lists of questions to be asked during the encounter. . . . The need to get specific information, to fill in the blanks in the mental and written forms, is very great. This may push physicians toward regarding their talk with patients as nonconversational" (1998:182). If different preconceptions by doctor and patient impede a successful encounter, both may feel frustrated and powerless in that situation. As I mentioned in chapter 3, the role allocated to patients in the biomedical framework also requires compliance with the treatment suggestions made by the medical specialist in order to regain health. In cases of domestic violence this predetermined patient role may pose a problem if women seemingly do not adhere to what doctors may expect of them or even advise them to do, that is, to leave their abusive partners.

Another important factor in the consultation frame is the way illness is perceived by both doctor and patient. Illness and disease can undoubtedly be located in a "natural framework," since they are usually caused by natural aggressors such as bacteria or viruses, which have a harmful impact on the physical condition of a person. In that sense, people are seen as being involuntarily exposed to disease, and they are not normally attributed an active role in the process of becoming ill. The role of the doctor as a health care professional is to help the individual patient who does not have the expertise to overcome the problem alone. Yet, to come back to the questions I posed at the outset of this book, what happens if the problem the patient presents in a consultation cannot be explained in terms of the biomedical model alone and hence cannot be remedied by merely prescribing medication? What if the "signs" have a psychosocial origin and the problem must therefore be interpreted and dealt with in a "social framework"? We must not forget that one of the perturbations of GPS is that even if they "fix" the damage, the patient might be hurt again. Agency becomes vital in this respect, since it entails questions concerning blame and responsibility. These questions must be considered against the wider background of medical ethics, which has traditionally been founded on three cornerstones: doctors' *decorum*, which includes politeness and respectfulness but also courage and resoluteness; *deontology*, which refers to doctors' duties and obligations; and *politic ethics*, which has to do with doctors' accountability to the wider community (Jonsen 2000). When patients' noncompliance with suggested treatment measures is perceived by doctors to infringe on their professional requirements, they may well feel frustrated and start to blame patients. O'Connor maintains that the "noncompliant" patient is considered "deviant, uncooperative, negligent, stubborn, ignorant, unreliable, or at the very least in default" (1995:174). This opinion "contributes to negative stereotyping and the damage that stereotyping always does, and tempts or allows health professionals to blame patients for not getting well" (O'Connor 1995:174). As I demonstrate below, stereotyping and blaming can also be found in the GPs' narratives in my sample.

Linguistically, agency can be dealt with in two interconnected ways: first, with regard to thematic roles (also referred to as theta roles) and, second, with regard to active/passive constructions. The theory of thematic structures, or, for short, theta theory, goes back to the early works of Gruber (1965), Fillmore (1968), and Jackendoff (1972), who proposed that each argument of the predicate (i.e., the subject or complement) carries a particular thematic role and that thematic functions are drawn from a limited universal set. The thematic roles that are of interest for this study are *agent/actor*, that is, the instigator of some action, and *patient/theme*, the entity that undergoes the effect of some action (Radford 1988:373). I henceforth use the Latin terms *agens* and *patiens* instead of the English "agent" and "patient," since the grammatical term "patient" could obviously cause some confusion in the context of doctor-patient interaction. The function of these two thematic roles can be illustrated with the following example:

> John hits Jill.

Grammatically speaking, the subject in this sentence is "John," and "Jill" is the direct object. In terms of thematic roles "John" is the *agens* and "Jill" is the *patiens* of the action expressed in the verb "hit." If we convert this sentence into its passive voice, the grammatical structure changes:

> Jill is hit by John.

Both arguments "Jill" and "John" maintain their thematic roles of *patiens* and *agens,* respectively, but their grammatical relations change: "Jill" is now subject, and "John" appears in the oblique case. In any passive construction either the *agens* can be left out completely and is thus removed from focus, or it can be added in a prepositional phrase with "by," which makes agency explicit and brings it back into focus. In the following analysis of the GPS' discourses I investigate how agency is linguistically constructed and what implications this can have for GPS' perceptions of and attitudes toward domestic violence victims.

Victims as Agents of Their Own Victimization

When the doctors in my sample spoke in general about victims of domestic violence, they frequently used passive constructions:

> 1. a. they**'ve been beaten up**
>   b. one or two middle-class people who *are abused*
>   c. they**'d been assaulted**
>   d. person who **is being victimized**
>   e. the last person I had in who'd been complaining of **being hit**
>   f. someone**'s been attacked**
>   g. she**'s been abused**
>   h. a lot of women **are abused** verbally
>   j. the girl that **got** her arm **broken**

In using passive constructions, which are often combined with the generalizing pronoun "they" or the impersonal noun phrases "someone" or "person," doctors present violence as agentless, that is, the male perpetrator is left out of the picture. Trinch also found in her study of Latinas' and legal helpers' abuse narratives that "the purpose of the passive construction is to deflect the importance of the agent" (2003:20). This might have to do with the fact that the GP often sees only the woman patient within the limited time span of the consultation, or the GP might be the partner's doctor as well and therefore be more concerned about issues of confidentiality. If this is true, however, it also reveals doctors' lack of interest in engaging more in the personal circumstances and background of patients and a reluctance to explore underlying problems further.

I must add here that the GPs in my sample did occasionally talk about perpetrators of violence and the possible reasons for their behavior, but this was mainly done in response to the following question: "Why, do you think, does domestic violence happen?" Patients, on the other hand, are quite literally assigned the role of *patiens*; that is, women victims are depicted as being passive, and, what is more, their gender remains unspecified. Even where active constructions are used, the violence spoken about often remains vague:

2. a. women come in with injuries that they**'ve sustained**
   b. there's lots of folk who **are involved** in domestic violence
   c. people who **have had** violent episodes
   d. women who **are experiencing** domestic violence
   e. **a final hitting out**
   f. **fights between partners**
   g. systematic torture a lot of women **go through**
   h. they seem to **have stumbled** from one abusive relationship to another
   i. I know a lot of women who just **continued to put themselves at risk**

In these examples the male perpetrator is as absent as in the passive sentences in (1) above. The violent incident is described, for example, in a gerund construction (2e) or in the extended noun phrase "fights between partners" (2f), where agency is equally distributed to both parties in a relationship. In examples (2a) to (2d) victims are assigned the thematic role of *patiens*, but they retain the subject position in the sentences, which implicitly makes them appear more active in relation to the verb. The last two examples, (2h) and (2i), provide the female victim with an agentive role. While in (2h) the verb "stumble" still implies somewhat helpless and involuntary movement, the verb phrase in (2i) clearly indicates deliberate action and thus agency on the part of the woman.

The attribution of agency to the victims is a striking and frequent theme that pervades to a greater or lesser extent all the interviews, regardless of whether the doctor was male or female. The following narrative told by a middle-aged male doctor from a city-center practice illustrates how doctors frame women linguistically as the agents of their own victimization. The narrative was told in response to the question: "Is there any case that is very vivid in your memory?"

Narrative 5

1. I had one particular [patient] who's, who is, you know, in her second or third abusive relationship, er,
2. and I, I just feel powerless, you know.
3. I mean this woman by choice has sought out yet another person.
4. Maybe not "sought out,"
5. I mean maybe it's that, er, her, her social, er, mix is with people who share that same, er, manner [?] to their previous partners.
6. You know, if they're all boozers and they all meet in the pub or whatever
7. then it's likely that she's gonna meet other people who, who are similar,
8. you know, in that we all tend to, um, find friendship with people who are or who have similarities.
9. So it's, it's maybe not so surprising.
10. But it's most surprising to me why people choose, er, to, to, to reenter, er, an arena of further physical violence, having got out of a previous one.
11. I find that really tough.

The first clause, which offers an orientation to the subsequent story, introduces the protagonist, who remains unspecified through the use of the indeterminate numeral "one" but who is then given special status through the adjective "particular," which makes this patient stand out from other female patients. Another interesting feature to note in this opening sentence is the switch from past tense, the most commonly used tense in narratives of personal experience (Labov 1997:400), to present tense. This indicates either that the case is still open and currently being dealt with by the doctor or that the present tense is used to underpin the universal validity of what is being said in this story. The fact that the opening sentence is immediately followed by a clause that functions as a first evaluative device ("I just feel powerless, you know") seems to reinforce the idea that the narrative initiated here serves the purpose of representing an exemplary case, and it underlines the narrator's opinion about this patient and her behavior.

In line 3 the GP elaborates on the reason why he feels "powerless" with regard to this patient: the woman "by choice has sought out yet another person" who is violent toward her. Significantly enough, the thematic structure and the active voice of the verb chosen here clearly attribute an agentive role to the woman. In other words, the patient deliberately looked for another violent partner. This notion of agency is emphasized even more through the insertion of the adverbial prepositional phrase "by choice" between subject and verb phrase, which implies again that the woman found an abusive partner by her own volition. The motif of choice is resumed in line 10 in the verb "choose." It is a motif that runs invariably through the GPs' responses in the interviews, as I discuss below.

The Negotiation of "Agency" in Narrative 5

Line 4 ("Maybe not 'sought out'") is very interesting in this narrative because it shows how interpersonal perception influences the way the interviewee formulates his response and thus underlines the notion of oral narratives as *socio-narratives*, that is, situated at the interface of linguistic, cognitive, and contextual factors (Herman 1999b). The fact that this GP uses the self-repair "Maybe not 'sought out,'" thereby questioning his own word choice, reveals a high level of self-monitoring in his speech. One may infer that the doctor was not entirely sure how I as a woman with a research interest in domestic violence would react to the wording of the preceding clause, which clearly presents the female victim in a fairly negative and critical light. The self-repair strategy mitigates the previous comment and ties in immediately with an attempt at further explication.

Lines 5 to 8 contain a sequence of clauses that can be interpreted as an explanatory sequence building up toward the main point of the story, namely, why women's seemingly irrational behavior can be explained to some extent but still remains something of a puzzle for the narrator: "I mean maybe it's that, er, her, her social, er, mix is with people who share that same, er, manner [?] to their previous partners. You know, if they're all boozers and they all meet in the pub or whatever then it's likely that she's gonna meet other people who, who are similar. You know, in that we all tend to, um, find friendship with people who are or who have similarities." A number of things are conspicuous in the scenario that the GP evokes in this sequence. First of all, we can find numerous discourse markers such as "I mean" and "you know" on the narrative context level of the interview frame. They are used to establish rapport between speaker and listener and also help interlocutors negotiate meaning and ensure mutual understanding (Schiffrin 1987). The GP clearly makes an effort here to convey to the interviewer his way of rationalizing the woman's strange life. The plausibility of this explanation, however, is indirectly called into question through the repetition of the adverbial "maybe" in lines 5 and 9, which puts the whole story in the hypothetical mode and presents it as the doctor's speculation about how this woman came to have another violent partner. In other words, the story the GP relates is more or less fictional because the doctor does not really know, apart from the limited knowledge he has of the woman through his practice work, how she leads her life. Nevertheless, the scenario he conjures up is very vivid. It is one that again reinforces the commonly held myths that domestic violence is mostly caused under the influence of alcohol and that it occurs predominantly in the lower social classes. Thus, the GP talks about the woman's "social mix," which is mainly with other "boozers" who "all meet in the pub." The stylistic incongruity between a very elaborate, formal style throughout most of the interview and a rather colloquial style expressed in the word "boozers" can be interpreted as the GP's attempt to evoke linguistically the social context of the scene presented here, the pub, but it also creates a sense of "otherness" and distance between the GP and "that kind of scene," as it were, since this lexical item does not really suit the overall interview register and therefore almost seems to convey a mocking tone. The emphasis on the idea of "two of a kind," which is repeated three times in the extended noun phrases "people who share that same manner," "people who are similar," and "people who have similarities," also gives the impression that this doctor does not have a high opinion of his patient. In fact, he puts her into the same category of people as her abusive partner. The logical connector "then" in line 7 invites the listener to the conclusion spelled out in line 9: maybe it is "not so surprising" after all that this woman is in another abusive relationship if she socializes with alcoholics.

Lines 10 and 11 form the final evaluation section, in which the GP states, contrary to his preceding explanations, that he cannot really understand his patient's behavior or indeed the behavior of any woman who falls victim to yet another abusive partner: "But it's most surprising to me why people choose, er, to, to, to reenter, er, an arena of further physical violence having got out of a previous one. I find that really tough." The GP resumes the motif of choice and attributes an agentive role to the victim with the verb "reenter," which implies that women deliberately find abusive men. The image of the "arena" is very interesting in this context, since it evokes associations with ancient amphitheaters where violence formed part of the daily entertainment. In this sense, the image indirectly conveys a sense of irony.

To sum up, not only does narrative 5 illustrate the way agency is constructed, but the detailed linguistic analysis also shows how the GP attempts to negotiate his viewpoint with the interviewer by applying the discursive strategies mentioned above.

Patient Noncompliance and Doctors' Helplessness

GPs' incredulity and powerlessness in view of the fact that women often return to their violent partners was one of the main themes running through the narratives. Although there have been a number of attempts to explain women's decision to stay,[2] no theory can adequately accommodate all the possibilities and provide a conclusive answer. As Schornstein puts it: "In working with victims, it is important to recognize that there are no pat answers to explain the responses of victims as a class. . . . Each victim is different, and she brings to the moment of crisis a life time of her own experiences that may affect her reaction and response to violence" (1997:54). The fact that some women stay with or return to their partners may thus be difficult for GPs to understand. The problem, I would argue, is not so much one of gender or of social class differences between doctor and patient as of divergent personal life experiences, which makes it difficult for doctors who may never have been victimized themselves to feel genuine empathy for their patients. In that sense, what Donald says about doctors' and patients' divergent experiences of illness is also true of the experience of domestic abuse: "Illness is a realm that the ill person *inhabits*, whereas disease categories are often quite crude maps that health professionals use to interpret the ill person's experience, from the other side of the wellness-illness divide" (1998:23, emphasis in original). If one considers that cases of domestic violence can be emotionally taxing for doctors, too, then it is not surprising that women's "noncompliance" with what, on the surface, seems to be the best solution for them (i.e., to leave their partners) can lead to GPs' frustration and a sense of helplessness (see also chapter 6). Let us have a brief look at another narrative that deals specifically with these feelings. Narrative 26 was related by a young female GP from a suburban practice.

Narrative 26

1. I mean I've got one in particular who,
2. her husband, um, is an alcoholic
3. and is abusive and aggressive towards her
4. and now towards her baby, er,
5. [he] use, you know, sort of uses her as a, as a weapon.
6. And she has tried to leave him
7. and has got an injunction against him
8. but then has changed her mind
9. and just gone back to him again.
10. And there's not much more I can do in that scenario really, which I find very difficult 'cause she's still upset about it and she's still affected by it so.

The Transmission of Emotions: Analysis of Narrative 26

Like narrative 3 presented at the beginning of this book, narrative 26 also centers around the woman's decision to stay with her partner, but it is less emotionally charged than narrative 3. The narrative starts with a fairly extensive orientation, which covers half of the entire narrative (lines 1 to 5). In this orientation section the interviewer is given information on the family situation, which is marked as current and habitual by the use of the simple present. The violent partner is classified as "alcoholic" (line 2), which is reminiscent of other narratives in the sample and reinforces the commonly held view that alcohol is often related to domestic violence. Furthermore, the woman's husband is described as "abusive and aggressive" (line 3) toward both his wife and her baby, and the violence is depicted in more detail in line 5: "sort of uses her as a, as a weapon." While the semantic roles of *agens* and *patiens* are clearly distributed to the husband as the acting figure and the wife and her baby as sufferers in the first half of the narrative, the roles are reversed at the beginning of the second half, where the woman becomes the social actor who takes action against her husband, the new *patiens*: "she has tried to leave him and has got an injunction against him" (lines 6 and 7). This sequence can be regarded as the complicating action of the narrative, which culminates in the turning point in line 8: "but then has changed her mind." As mentioned earlier, the logical connector "but" expresses opposing action (Schiffrin 1987), and in this case the woman's change of mind is contrasted with her previously active behavior. The patient's lack of responsible and "reasonable" action finally results in her return to her husband: "and just gone back to him again" (line 9). The locative adjunct "to him" is grammatically redundant in this sentence but is used to emphasize the target of the woman's movement, of which the GP did not approve, as she admitted after she had finished her narrative: "You just wish you could say: 'Right, just leave him!'"

What is most interesting in this narrative is the fact that there does not seem to be any space for the GP. While semantic roles are allocated to all members of the family, the family doctor is left out of the picture, which in a way epitomizes the marginal role the GP sees for herself and even openly addresses at the end of the narrative: "there's not much more I can do in that scenario really" (line 10). Although the narrative as such is unemotional in its tone, the GP finally mentions feelings when she says that she finds it "very difficult" (line 10) because the patient is "still upset about it and she's still affected by it" (line 10). The parallel structure in the last two subordinate clauses underlines the patient's emotional state, which also affects the doctor. Nevertheless, the "message" that is conveyed does not focus on the patient's background and possible reasons for why she stays with her partner but on the fact that she went back and that this makes it impossible for the doctor to take further measures. As for narrative 3, one can argue that, if this rather undifferentiated narrative about a woman's return to her violent partner becomes narrative memory that can be consulted in the future, then this might preclude the storage and implementation of more detailed narratives that might introduce the woman's perspective, on the one hand, and provide space for doctors' agency, on the other.

The Motif of Choice and GPs' Lack of Comprehension

Narratives 5 and 26 seem to reconstruct agency to the disadvantage of the patients and thus reveal the doctors' lack of understanding for why their patients stay in a violent relationship. Viewed against the background of domestic violence research, most of the interviews appear to be marked by this lack of comprehension. Although the GPs sometimes tried to explain the behavior of victims in terms of financial dependence and the women's concerns about their families, the overall tenor of their responses makes it clear that battered women are often implicitly blamed for being victims. The following quotes give an idea of the range of comments made by the GPs in my sample (note that the comments presented in [4] were made by female doctors).

> 3. a. **Why** should they put up with it, you know, if they've got an **alternative,** yeah, and get out? Er, but of course [you get all those who] sometimes return to it, er, or on occasions, er, where **by genetic disposition** make the **unfortunate mistake of picking another one** violent partner in a second or possibly the third relationship.

> b. There maybe is a mechanism for teaching women not to accept that sort of behavior or, er, to **unlearn it.** It's **part of their culture.**

> c. At the end of the day, well, people can be trapped in [?] situations, and if you've got kiddies and stuff **they might feel more obligated to carry on getting thumped** or whatever, I don't know.

> d. I suppose, it's, er, they're even sort of, a degree of **sadomasochism,** that some people actually **like being beaten up,** er.

> e. **Certain people attract that,** they're just, because they **put up less resistance** and, er, and that again makes it more difficult to just be up front because being up front again takes courage, which is what they don't have in the first place. So, it's a bit of a vicious cycle, I suppose.

> 4. a. Er, I think a lot of it is 'cause **the women allow it to happen.** They feel, er, **dependent** on, on individuals. Er, I think because they don't have that much, er, self-esteem herself [sic], awareness.

b. You know, I feel it's so, it's, it's so wrong that somebody can allow viol—
— or, somebody can be violent to somebody else and other peo——,
and then . . . **the victim can allow her- or himself to be
victimized.**

c. Er, I mean, what we see is, women can be treated dreadfully by
men. I see a lot of that, not just violence but, you know, just, well,
allow themselves to become doormats and get pregnant over and
over again, you know, whatever, **get a poorer image of themselves**
and perhaps, yeah. So, um, **downtrodden,** yeah, so.

d. I mean, sometimes you just think people are rea——, **being really
silly,** you know, they've been beaten near to death on ten occasions
and **still go back. I mean, what can you do? What can you do?**

A number of the highlighted lexical items and phrases in the text are worthy of
comment. Example (3a) starts with a question related to the one mentioned at
the outset of this chapter, "Why do they stay?": "Why should they put up with
it?" The modal auxiliary "should" expresses obligation, and its use here indicates that the GP does not understand why women might feel compelled to accept violence. The noun "alternative" implies that women have choices, a theme
that runs consistently through the interviews. The logical conclusion from that
assumption is that if a woman suffers domestic violence it is because she has decided to take up the victim role, which, hence, is her own fault, as can be seen in
the statements made in (4a) to (4c): "the women allow it to happen," "the victim can allow her- or himself to be victimized," "allow themselves to become
doormats." Example (4b) is especially interesting linguistically, since it combines the verb "allow," which assigns the role of *agens* to its subject, "victim,"
with the passive construction "being victimized." Women are paradoxically depicted as agents of what is otherwise seen as an agentless process, so one finds
either agentless victimization or agency on the victim's part.

The linguistic reconstruction of victims as having choices can have far-reaching consequences, as research conducted by Ehrlich (1999, 2001) demonstrates.
Ehrlich (1999) discusses in her article on the representation of sexual assault
the language used in a university sexual harassment tribunal. She shows how
the questions two of the tribunal members asked presupposed the deficiency of
the complainants' signals of resistance. This alleged lack of resistance was then

interpreted as tantamount to consent, although both female victims characterized their experience as assault. One of the strategies the tribunal members
used was to present the victims as having had "options" and thereby to imply
their inaction. They could have left the room, for example, or could have told
the offender to stop his advances. The women's fear was minimized. Ehrlich
argues that the tribunal members constructed an interpretive frame in which
the female victims were "represented as having exercised some agency, or even
having chosen to engage in the sexual activities" (1999:245). At the beginning of
this chapter I discussed what Goffman (1974) calls "social frameworks," whereby
victims are reconstructed as actors with a right to self-determination, legal com-
petence, and moral obligations. Ehrlich, however, demonstrates that this view
of victims neglects other factors such as fear and power relations between men
and women: "That is, constructing complainants as freely-choosing, autono-
mous individuals, as legal doctrine does, precludes a consideration of the material conditions under which their consent is 'meaningful': conditions in which
the victims' fear and paralysis (and not their minds) can be 'dominant and
controlling,' given the unequal power dynamics that potentially characterize
male/female relations in situations of unwanted sexual aggression" (2001:92).
Similarly, the GPs in my sample indirectly present victims of domestic violence
as inactive and therefore responsible for their situation. At the same time, victims are reconstructed as "deviant." Williamson contends: "Producing a notion
that women who experience domestic violence should leave violent relationships, when there already exists a very powerful social discourse which advocates that women should keep relationships and families very firmly together,
adds to those cultural myths which allow individuals both personally and professionally within all agencies to perceive women within violent relationships
as in some way deviant or stigmatised in themselves" (2000:28).

Redefining Battered Women as the "Deviant Other"

Other explanations proposed by some of the doctors clearly stigmatize victims
as displaying a weak character or deviant behavior; for example, women choose
violent partners due to their "genetic disposition" (3a) or because "it's part of
their culture" (3b). Female victims are framed as "victim types," "vulnerable
individuals," and "dependent women" who are possibly "less intelligent than
their husband." They might have a tendency toward "sadomasochism" (3d), or

violence occurs because "certain people attract that" (3d). One male GP nearing retirement commented:

> 5. Um, for a start, who do you treat? Er, **does the woman have a
> problem,** you know, because she's being beaten up? Is that not a re-
> sult of being beaten up or **does she have a problem** that perhaps, er,
> meshes with her partner's problem, um, I don't know.

This doctor presents domestic abuse as a result of a "problem" both in the male
perpetrator and in the victim. The GP thus insinuates that being a victim of violence presupposes an "abnormality" of some sort in the woman's character or
psychological disposition. Similarly, another middle-aged male GP suggested
"anything from counselling services to, er, Cornhill Hospital for psychiatric
or psychological assessment" as possible solutions, thereby implying that the
woman, not her perpetrator, has a psychological problem.[3] A number of GPs
mentioned alcohol as one common cause for the occurrence of violence, and one
middle-aged male GP presented a narrative about a couple where both partners
are alcoholics (narrative 29). This kind of response underpins the following assumption made by Kurz and Stark: "We speculate that clinicians make an 'implicit diagnosis' of abuse in which psychosocial sequelae such as alcoholism or
depression are viewed as its cause and where the woman—not her assailant or
his violence—is seen as 'sick'" (1990:259–60). Although the term "sick" is not
necessarily used in a purely medical sense, the redefinition of victims as alcoholics and depressed or even mentally disturbed women in a way legitimizes
the women's role as patients and thus warrants treatment. The treatment battered women are offered is often misled, however, because it tackles physical
symptoms rather than the violence itself, as Bograd's (1987) and Williamson's
(2000) studies demonstrate.

Implicit Blame Culture and Stigmatizing Discourses

It is interesting that especially male GPs seem to construct victims of domestic violence as the "deviant other": "other" not only in terms of gender but also
in terms of irrational behavior for which they cannot easily find an explanation. And yet even some of the responses given by the female GPs do not necessarily show greater understanding. The highly judgmental and trivializing
verb phrase "being really silly" in (4d) and the "doormat" metaphor in (4c)

indicate disapproval that women might sense when they go to see their GP. Loseke and Cahill (1984) and Lamb (1999) maintain that professionals often define victims of abuse in a discrediting manner and thus indirectly victimize women further. As Williamson's research also shows, women frequently encounter in medical settings "the abusive social discourse of domestic violence which blames women for the abuse they experience" (2000:49). One woman in Williamson's sample, Helena, tells the interviewer how a nurse implied that she had provoked violence in her abusive partner: "a . . . nurse said to me, 'What did you do to upset him?'" (2000:49). Even though accusations are not made as directly and openly by the GPs in my sample, the pattern that emerges from the GPs' responses indicates a (possibly unconscious) blame culture by which women are held responsible for their situation.

The GPs' readiness to indirectly blame the victim herself is alarming. However, it is not a phenomenon that is unique to health care professionals, as, for example, Meyers's (1997) study of the representation of violence against women in the news media shows. I will come back to this point in my final chapter. The stigmatization of victims, whether conscious or unconscious, can be harmful in a consultation when a woman experiencing violence senses the GP's resistance and consequently feels inhibited from opening up. For this reason it is important to uncover the conceptual frames doctors apply to domestic violence with regard to women's agency and, moreover, to unravel the underlying linguistic mechanisms by which these frames are set up. It is equally important, however, to investigate how doctors present agency as far as their own professional role is concerned.

"You just can't fix it for them": Modals and the Delegation of Responsibility

In the previous chapter I considered the ways GPs conceptualize domestic violence as a social rather than a medical problem and therefore deflect responsibility from themselves. Here I complement this discussion by looking at a similar strategy related to the construction of victims. Victims are implicitly interpreted within a social framework in which they are given a role that entails free will and decision making as well as a legal and moral obligation to take responsibility. This way of conceptualizing victims of domestic violence places them outside the sphere of intervention by the doctor, and, consequently, GPs have a valid argument for denying agency to themselves. In other words, if the victim does not take measures to change her life, it is not the GP's place to do anything about it either. The following comments made by the GPs in my sample reveal this strategy of distancing:

6. a. There's nothing, a lot of that is **within the woman's own hand.** I just try and give her the confidence and try to empower her, but **she should take some sort of action.**

b. I can't get too involved in that. There are too many things going on. Er, but people, I guess, have some **responsibility to themselves** and their own actions.

c. You can't make somebody leave somebody, it's **not your responsibility.** People **have to make their own decisions.**

d. **Patients have choices** themselves or, you know, they can get in touch with the police or social work.

e. You often do feel that your, **your hands are a bit tied** 'cause you can't, y——you can't initiate, er, sort of appropriate steps for them. **They've got to actually be willing** to do it.

f. At the end of the day **it's the woman that decides.**

g. And you can advise, you can get the health visitor involved, they can see Citizens Advice, they can do all these things but **unless they want to do it, they won't do it,** you know.

h. And you can say to them and say to them and say to them and they won't want to change it. You just say: **"Well, that's their lot."**

i. I think it's very much **up to the patient** or, what they want to do about it.

j. But I think, I think **they've got to decide** what to, what to do about it themselves.

The responses are strikingly similar (again, note that the comments presented in [6f] through [6j] were made by female doctors). A common denominator of all these responses is the theme of choice and the women's responsibility to make decisions themselves. The modal auxiliary "should" in (6a) ("she should take some sort of action") and the quasi-modal "have got to" in (6c) ("People have to make their own decisions"), (6e) ("They've got to actually be willing to do it"), and (6j) ("they've got to decide what to do") are significant in this respect, since they imply not only the women's choices in making decisions but in fact their obligation to do so. This attitude makes it easier for a GP to distance himself or herself from a patient's problem and to avoid a feeling of frustration if the patient does not accept his or her advice, as we can see in (6h): it is "their lot," not the doctor's.

Occasionally, GPs expressed the concern that some patients might regard open questions about domestic abuse posed by their GP as intrusive. Interestingly enough, this point is mostly elaborated through notions of "I" and "other"; that is, the patient is again reconstructed as an individual on the other side of the doctor-patient divide. The following statements illustrate this point:

> 7. a. **I can't impose the way that I choose to live my life** and the principles and moral-ethical, er, code that I use to order my life. I can't impose that on somebody else.

> b. **You can never tell people what to do.** You can perhaps let them tell their story and, er, explore their options, point them in directions where they can get help.

> c. **You can't expect your values and what you think you would do** to follow on to each individual.

> d. You feel like you want to empower them to do something but, again, **we can't put our, you know, aspects onto them** and it's, it's, I think you've, you've got to try and be clinical in some respects for them so that you don't, you don't become too emotive.

> e. I think **it's not your place to say, "Well, you should leave him,"** but, er, people have very complex reasons for staying together, I think, and you, **I don't think you should be intervening in that too much.**

In (7a), (7c), and (7d) the GPs talk about their own lives, values, and expectations, which they cannot impose on the lives of their patients. The predominant modal auxiliary used in this context is "can" combined with a negative marker such as "not" or "never." It implies the impossibility of the action described and, moreover, the speaker's feeling about the inappropriateness of such action and, consequently, his or her moral obligation not to take action. Furthermore, it is interesting to see that in most cases GPs choose the generic pronoun "you," thereby generalizing the moral dilemma they present and, at the same time, keeping it at a distance. Intervention or action on the part of the GP is seen as potentially intrusive and therefore unacceptable. One solution to this dilemma is to delegate the responsibility for dealing with the case to other agencies, as is indicated in (7b): the GP can "point them in directions where they can get help." This phrase implies that help is not available from the GP but from other sources that are spatially distant.

Summary

As this chapter shows, agency is a complex issue when considering domestic violence cases. While victims of violence are often framed as passive and helpless, cultural discourses on violence also present women as agents of their own victimization in the sense that they do not take action and leave their partners, for example. An insurmountable paradox is thus created that puzzles doctors and other people alike. Agency also becomes crucial for the assignment of the patient role. While patients are usually regarded as suffering involuntarily from an illness, they are also expected to comply with the expert knowledge and recommendations of doctors and thus to actively assume their patient role. In cases of domestic violence, where women may decide to go back to their partners, this patient role is not fulfilled in the sense of the biomedical model and may thus lead to GPs' frustration and resignation. Perhaps one way of getting around this dilemma is for doctors to accept that in many cases their task can only be limited to the role of witness and listener, to validating women's stories, and to having the necessary help resources at hand when required. As I show in the next chapter, however, doctors' readiness to help also depends on how seriously they take cases of domestic violence and what status domestic violence has amidst a whole range of other health issues. The following chapter deals with evaluation in the GPs' narratives or, in other words, with what the GPs deemed noteworthy and tellable in the stories they related.

8. Evaluating Abuse

Storied Knowledge and Salient Facts

Evaluation is "that part of the narrative which reveals the attitude of the narrator towards the narrative by emphasizing the relative importance of some narrative units as compared to others" (Labov and Waletzky 1967:37). Evaluative devices in a story signal to the listener that the narrated event is in some way unusual and that it is therefore worth telling, or, in Labov's words: "Evaluative devices say to us: this was terrifying, dangerous, weird, wild, crazy; or amusing, hilarious, wonderful; more generally, that it was strange, uncommon, or unusual—that is, worth reporting" (1972a:371). Evaluation in narratives answers the questions, What is the point of this story? Why does the narrator want to tell this story? In a sense, then, a speaker justifies to other interlocutors his or her telling a particular story by adding evaluation. In his 1997 article Labov redefines evaluation within the framework of what he calls "Sack's Assignment Theorem" (1997:405), namely with regard to turn-taking rules. He points out that "telling a narrative requires a person to occupy more social space than in other conversational exchanges—to hold the floor longer—and the narrative must carry enough interest for the audience to justify this action" (Labov 1997:404–5). Thus, evaluation comes to be viewed in more technical terms as a device for justifying "the automatic reassignment of speaker role to the narrator" (Labov 1997:406). Consequently, speakers have to decide to report the "most reportable event" before they embark on constructing a narrative, which then includes the ordering of this most reportable event in a logical and meaningful way within a series of other events. Speakers must, in a way, justify their telling of a story by making this story sound interesting and relevant in the given context. Norrick observes for storytelling in conversational discourse: "Since conversationalists tend to expect topical talk, stories on new topics routinely exhibit prefaces constructed to sell them as particularly interesting. Highly evaluative and emotionally loaded words and phrases fill this need" (2000:108). At the same time, a speaker gives away his or her personal feelings, thoughts, and attitudes toward the related story or some aspect of it.

In the interview situation the turn-taking mechanism underlying the gaining and yielding of the floor is less compelling, since the interviewee is automatically given more time to elaborate on a topic. That is, competition for the floor is less marked in interviews, and, consequently, one may assume that the telling of a story does not necessarily have to be based on considerations of the story being "reportable" or exciting. On the other hand, however, narratives are nonetheless expected to be to the point in a specific discursive situation. This is even more true if the narrative has been elicited through a question posed by an interviewer. I want to caution here against the assumption that some events can be considered reportable in their own right. Rather, I would argue that reportability is also socially constructed; that is, there are cultural expectations as to what counts as "interesting" or "reportable" elements of a story. Moreover, reportability is constructed and negotiated by speakers during storytelling. In other words, it emerges out of a specific narrative situation in which narrators signal reportable events through linguistic cues. The various types of evaluation are accompanied by a number of linguistic devices. Labov's (1972a) conceptual starting point is the assumption that there is a basic "narrative syntax" along which all oral narratives are created. This narrative syntax contains the following eight elements (adapted from Labov 1972a:376):

1. Conjunctions, including temporals: "so," "and," "but," "then"
2. Simple subjects such as pronouns and proper names
3. An underlying auxiliary that is a simple past tense marker and is incorporated in the verb; no member of the auxiliary appears in the surface structure except in the occasional progressive form in the orientation section and in quasi modals such as "start," "begin," "keep," "used to," and "want"
4. Preterit verbs, with adverbial particles such as "up," "over," "down"
5. Complements of varying complexity
6. Manner of instrumental adverbials
7. Locative adverbials
8. Temporal adverbials and comitative clauses

Technically speaking, evaluative devices generally complicate this basic narrative syntax by deviating from it.

As I mentioned in chapter 3, twelve of the narratives the GPs related in the interviews were interviewer initiated, while twenty-four narratives can be classified as "spontaneous." Spontaneous narratives are probably more interesting as far as evaluative function is concerned, because they are obviously related on the narrator's own initiative and thus reveal something about the narrator's aim in telling a particular story. As Daiute and Nelson point out: "Scripts, representing *what happens* in general, do not require an internal evaluative component. Stories, however, whether fictional or personal narratives, need a point of view that incorporates an evaluative component implicitly or explicitly. What happened was triumphant or tragic, surprising, gratifying, or disappointing" (1997:208, emphasis in original). Therefore, the questions that arise for narrative analysis are, What is the purpose or function of a narrative in a given discursive context? What does that indicate with regard to the narrator's viewpoint relative to the topic under discussion? In this chapter I investigate why the doctors related the particular stories they told me in the interviews and not others; what was especially memorable about these events; and, finally, what this indicates with regard to the GPs' perception of domestic violence in general.

Evaluation and GPs' Storied Knowledge of Domestic Violence

I start by comparing two narratives that were elicited in response to explicit questions I asked during the interview. Narrative 32 was told by a young female GP in a practice bordering on the city center, and narrative 15 was told by a late-middle-aged male doctor in a student health practice.

Narrative 32

J: Right, okay, but can you tell me a bit about the experiences you've had?

1. Um, so, I suppose, there was one girl in particular
2. I remember her being really quite a hard thing for me.
3. She was always at the surgery, minor, usually minor, minor complaints
4. or she'd drag along her little boy
5. and it'd be something very minor with him, um,

6. and they were here all the time
7. and then, one day, basically she admitted that, you know,
8. I'd actually visited her at home as well, in the presence of this very "loving" in inverted commas boyfriend
9. and then one day she admitted to me that he'd been abusing her for ^ years
10. but her son was out of, as a result of a rape,
11. and it was just horrendous.
12. Now, since that has come up I have never, I see her once a year.
13. So, in the long run, I've saved a lot of time
14. and she's perhaps, she's got rid of the boyfriend, which was the real cure,
15. there was nothing medical I could do for her, um,
16. but that really sticks in my mind, that case.

Narrative 15

J: Is there any case that's particularly vivid in your memory?
1. There was one girl, yeah, that was pinned to a wall and had her head bashed in, and by someone, er, another student, um,
2. and she was terrified
3. and it definitely affected her in a bad way,
4. I mean, she, um, she left [?]
5. and the person that assaulted her, that was an atrocious sight.
6. She was bigger than me,
7. I remember that.
8. That's the most, that's the only one that has been in the last seven years where there was a real problem, you know, where there was a, a difficult outcome, if you like.
9. The rest, they were all minor.

General Analysis of Narrative 32

Narrative 32 begins with information on the person involved in the story: "one girl": "Um, so, I suppose there was one girl in particular." It is interesting that this doctor refers to her obviously grown-up patient and mother of a little boy as "girl." Since this GP classified all the patients she spoke about in the interview as "girls," it might be inferred that she was not conscious of age. At the same time, however, "girls" conjures up female patients who suffer domestic violence as immature women who are perhaps too weak to deal with their problem. Line 2 is the first evaluative clause in the narrative that states why the doctor remembers this particular patient and why she therefore considers this story worth telling: "I remember her being really quite a hard thing for me." The attributive adjective "hard," which is doubly strengthened by the preceding intensifying adverbs "really" and "quite," signals to the listener that this case is memorable because it was a difficult case for the doctor. The evaluation is made more explicit in the very last clause of the narrative, where the doctor actually says: "that really sticks in my mind, that case." Moreover, the verb in the present tense clearly marks the end of the narrative and the narrator's return to the present situation, that is, the interview frame. In this sense line 16 can be regarded as part of the coda, which starts in line 12 with the temporal adverb "now" ("Now, since that has come up") and which is only interrupted in lines 14 and 15, where the narrative is resumed to explain what the outcome of the story was: "she's got rid of the boyfriend, which was the real cure, there was nothing medical I could do for her." Line 15 is interesting as far as evaluative devices are concerned, because the clause is part of the narrative proper, indicated by the past tense, but at the same time it also indicates to the listener how the narrator evaluates the case in retrospect: there was "nothing medical" the doctor could do for her patient. In Labov's terminology negatives function as *comparators* in the sense that they "compare the events which did occur to those which did not occur" (1972a:381). The claim that doctors cannot do much for patients who suffer domestic violence because domestic violence is not, strictly speaking, a medical problem is a major theme that runs through almost all the interviews I conducted, as I discussed in chapter 6.

Lines 3 to 6 contain a sequence of short clauses that form the complicating action: "She was always at the surgery, minor, usually minor, minor complaints or she'd drag along her little boy and it'd be something very minor with him, um, and they were here all the time." At first glance the action expressed in these clauses seems rather trivial and hardly worth telling. Many people go to see their doctor frequently and often for minor problems. There is nothing unusual about the events presented here. What makes this sequence interesting within the narrative, however, is the fact that the narrator implies a *rea-*

son for these events. By emphasizing the repetitive and regular nature of this patient's visits through the modal auxiliary "would" and through the temporal adverbials "always" and "all the time," which quantify the occurrence, the doctor suggests that her patient came on purpose, namely, because she suffered domestic violence and because she was seeking help. Bower terms this type of clause a "deliberative action construct" (DAC), that is, it is a clause that "allow[s] us to see in some detail how referential and evaluative components at multiple levels in the complicating action section operate to communicate both action and meaning" (1997:57). Since the repetitiveness of the narrated event is linguistically enacted in this sequence of clauses and also in the repetition of the evaluative adjective "minor," the whole complicating action sequence can be regarded as a device for building up suspense. Ironically, this point does not seem to hold if one considers that I as the listener anticipated the outcome of the story, since the interview was obviously on domestic violence, and that "suspense" therefore did not center around the question "What happened in the end?" but rather "How did it all come about?" The fact that this doctor still uses DACs points to the fact that, at least in the Western tradition, people have an inherent notion that building up suspense is an essential element in the narrative repertoire.

The resolution section is introduced in line 7: "and then, one day, basically she admitted that." It is clearly set off from the complicating action section by the temporal connector "then" and by the fact that the unspecified time scale of the repetitive action in lines 3 to 7 is now brought to a stop, "one day." The content of the resolution section refers to the patient's admission that her boyfriend "had been abusing her," a lengthy and ongoing ordeal that is emphasized by the progressive verb form and the phonetically stressed temporal adverb "for years" in line 9. The final resolution, however, is again suspended by the insertion of the clause in line 8, which should be part of the complicating action section but has been extracted and shifted back within the narrative in order to postpone the content of what the woman actually admitted to: "I'd actually visited her at home as well, in the presence of this very 'loving' in inverted commas boyfriend." This clause also receives evaluative force, since the doctor reconsiders events of the past in the light of her present knowledge. The "very loving boyfriend" was not really a loving boyfriend at all, as is indicated by the linguistic gesture "in inverted commas," but the doctor did not discover the truth until later. For this reason, the woman's disclosure of domestic violence, the impact of which is magnified through the additional disclosure of the rape story in line 10 ("but her son was out of, as a result of rape"), came as a shock to the doctor and is duly commented upon in line 11: "it was just horrendous." The *reportable event* in this narrative is therefore not the fact that the woman had been abused but that it took the doctor such a long time to find out what was going on.

General Analysis of Narrative 15

Let us now turn to the second narrative to see in what way it differs from narrative 32. Narrative 15 opens with a miniorientation section that introduces the protagonist, again "one girl," but it then moves immediately to the events and even the outcome of these events in the case described: "There was one girl, yeah, that was pinned to a wall and had her head bashed in, and by someone, er, another student." In contrast to narrative 32 there is no elaborate complicating action sequence, but the listener is thrust right in the middle of the story, a story that strikes us as being particularly shocking through its vivid description of a high degree of violence. Interestingly enough, the violent action is presented in a relative clause that depends syntactically on the noun phrase "one girl" and that has the function of further specifying this noun phrase. It is unusual that reportable events are put into a subordinate clause, which normally carries less semantic weight than a main clause. This discrepancy between narrated event and narrative presentation indicates two things: first, the doctor who told me this story was reflecting on this case in retrospect and was therefore no longer emotionally involved; second, he deliberately tried to appear unaffected in order to deepen the shocking effect of these events. Since this GP did not comply with the standard model of a narrative script in the Labovian sense, the immediate presentation of the resolution section came as a surprise for me as a listener and consequently caused me to be rather taken aback. The affirmative interjection "yeah" links the narrative to the interview situation. It could be interpreted as either an expression of the doctor's recalling the story to himself ("Yes, I remember this case") or as a signal to the listener that this is a story worth listening to ("Yes, I can tell you a story that will interest you"). The latter interpretation would ascribe evaluative force to this interjection.

The violent action described in line 1 is conveyed in a passive construction. This phenomenon occurs throughout my interviews, as I demonstrated in chapter 7, and normally the passive construction is used to cut the male perpetrator out of the picture. Considering the fact that around 85 percent of passive constructions in English are agentless (Celce-Murcia and Larsen-Freeman 1983:225), that is, the focus is on the action rather than on the agent, instances where the agent is made explicit are even more remarkable. In this clause the perpetrator is explicitly mentioned and, moreover, the presence of a violent agent is emphasized by the addition of the prepositional phrase "by someone," which is followed by the explanatory apposition "another student." Thus, the listener's attention is automatically drawn to this agent. This is done for a purpose that becomes clear in lines 5 and 6 after a couple of explanatory clauses depicting the emotional state of the victim in lines 2 and 3 ("and she was terrified and it definitely affected her in a bad way") and a very brief summary of the outcome of the story in line 4 ("I mean, she, um, she left"). Lines 5 and 6 contain a description of the perpetrator that is fairly lengthy in comparison with the overall narrative: "and the person that assaulted her, that was an atrocious sight. She was bigger than me." Again, the focus lies on the perpetrator, as can be seen in the left dislocation of the subject, which is taken up again through the depersonalizing demonstrative pronoun "that." What is unusual about this violent agent is conveyed to the listener in the judgmental adjective "atrocious" in line 5 and the comparator in line 6: "She was bigger than me." Not only is the perpetrator female, which deviates from the fact that domestic abuse is overwhelmingly perpetrated by men on women, but this female student is also extraordinary in that she is very big, indeed bigger than a man, as the doctor emphasizes.

The evaluative clause in line 7 sums up in the *verbum putandi* "remember" ("I remember that") why this case is worth telling or, in other words, why it is a reportable event, namely, because the violent agent was such a memorable person and because the visible result of this violence was gruesome. This evaluation is made more explicit in line 8, which contains a complex construction with the main clause and three subsequent relative clauses that depend on the noun phrase "the only one": "That's the most, that's the only one that has been in the last seven years where there was a real problem, you know, where there was a, a difficult outcome." The unusual nature of this case is already anticipated in the use of the superlative "most" and the intensifier "only" and is reinforced in the relative clauses that are introduced by the interrogative pronoun "where." The parallel structure of these relative clauses suggests an equation of the noun phrases "a real problem" and "a difficult outcome" and thus also implies the following logical connection: only if there is a difficult outcome can a case be considered a real problem. This view is confirmed in line 9, where the doctor classifies all other cases of domestic violence that he has seen as being "minor," in other words, not worth telling: "The rest, they were all minor." One may assume that those cases were also not worth memorizing in greater detail and have consequently failed to become part of the GP's narrative knowledge of domestic violence.

A Comparison of Narratives 32 and 15 Regarding Evaluation

If we compare the narrative structures and particularly the evaluative devices in these two narratives, it becomes clear that the two GPs apply rather different discursive strategies in order to interest the interviewer in what they have to say. The first GP follows largely the narrative model as outlined in Labov and Waletzky (1967). She uses DACs and the intermingling of complicating action and resolution in order to create suspense and then reconsiders the whole case in retrospect in a lengthy coda. Similarly, the second GP reflects the case he talks about from his present-day position. The GP's attitude in narrative 15, however, appears to be much more detached and unaffected, which is revealed in the lack of involvement in the narrative mode. Thus, the second GP does not use a sequence of simple narrative clauses in order to build up suspense in a complicating action sequence; instead, he presents a contracted version of the events by jumping straight in, as it were. I have interpreted this technique as a device for deepening the shocking effect of the violent story. This reminds us of the writing style found in tabloid journalism: detailed depictions of violent action that aim to shock people, a description of the emotional state of the victim, and a judgmental presentation of the perpetrator.

The two narratives also differ considerably in their *evaluation*. The evaluative devices in the first narrative indicate that the GP sees the point of telling her story not so much in the violent situation as such but more in the fact that she as a doctor failed to realize, over a lengthy period of time, what was really going on. The case as such is not remarkable in the sense that this kind of violence occurs on a daily basis in many families, but it has been made remarkable and indeed memorable in this GP's rendition of that case. Narrative 15 is different in that it already depicts a rather unusual or extreme case of violence where the doctor had to face serious medical consequences resulting from it. The evaluative devices the second GP applies in his narrative explicitly suggest that this case has in fact only become memorable *because of* the high degree of violence involved and *because of* the unusual perpetrator of this violence, a big female student. Recall that Labov and Waletzky defined evaluation as the part of a story that shows the narrator's attitude toward the story "by emphasizing the relative importance of some narrative units as compared to others" (1967:37). According to this definition, it appears that the first GP emphasizes silence and secrecy, whereas the second GP focuses on factual evidence in the form of physical signs of abuse. While the first GP generally evaluates domestic violence as a "hard" case for GPs because it is not easy to discover, the second GP seems to consider as serious only those cases in which there is a difficult physical outcome. In fact, this GP said explicitly later in the interview that none of the other cases he had had "stood out in the sense that they didn't, you know, bother me a lot." Hence, following Schank's (1990) reflections on the storage of stories in memory, these other cases were perhaps not stored as detailed narratives in the memorized stock of cases in this GP's knowledge base and will therefore not be as readily available as a resource for future reference when the next patient suffering domestic violence walks into his practice. Moreover, the provision of help may be measured against what "type" of case the GP is faced with, that is, whether doctors deem a case "serious" or not. These issues will be explored in the following section.

Reportable Events, Memory, and Stereotypes

Many of the thirty-six narratives that the doctors produced during the interviews followed the pattern of the second narrative in that they presented rather extraordinary incidents of domestic violence or unusual encounters with patients suffering domestic violence. Doctors presented, for example, scenarios where domestic violence occurred because both partners had a drinking problem or because the woman was schizophrenic and thus became an easier target for her abusive partner. Other cases involved the victim's attempt at suicide or a fatal outcome. It is important to stress that the physicians' gender did not really play a role in the way domestic violence cases were depicted. Both male and female GPs conjured up approximately the same type of unusual scenario, and even the wording overlaps sometimes. Thus, victims were depicted as being "pinned to a wall," or perpetrators were presented as "going out and getting drunk on a Friday night." Individual variations can be noticed to the extent that male GPs tended to dramatize cases by bluntly presenting a high degree of violence. Thus, one middle-aged doctor in a suburban practice remembered an alcohol-related case where the husband "didn't realize that she was dead until he sobered up and she had the head in the fireplace."

The fact that the narratives related unusual events can to some extent be explained in terms of cultural expectations surrounding the narrative frame. In our culture stories are usually exciting or extraordinary because that is required of "good" stories. In that sense the doctors probably volunteered narratives of this type because they assumed that that was what I as the interviewer expected to hear. Viewed against the backdrop of Bruner's (1986, 1991) and Schank's (1990) theories, the GPs' narratives can also be interpreted as indicating that mostly unusual cases have become part of the doctors' "storied" knowledge about domestic violence, whereas the more common cases may not have been labeled and stored in memory for later retrieval. This would also mean that cultural myths and clichés are perpetuated through the GPs' discourses. To follow up this assumption, let us consider another narrative. One older male GP related a story about a patient who had sadomasochistic tendencies and actually enjoyed being beaten up by her husband. Significantly, this story was unelicited by me, the interviewer, and was related in the context of a discussion of reasons for domestic violence.

Narrative 23

1. I suppose, it's, er, they're even sort of, a degree of sadomasochism, that some people actually like being beaten up, er, [?].

2. I mean I had a, a, I mean a patient many years ago

3. and she, I mean she used to come in and reg——, regale us with the, the most bizarre and, er, tales of terrible sadomastics, masochistic stuff and,

4. but she stayed with her husband for ten years, you know, um, er,

5. it was, um, you know, it, it was, it was almost sort of schizoid that, you know, she was,

   6. she'd sit there
   7. and say, "He's doing this, that, and the other," you know,
   8. "[took] me and beat me up"
   9. and "Why don't you leave?"
   10. "Oh, I can't leave!" [laughs], you know.

General Analysis of Narrative 23

The narrative starts with an abstract that introduces the topic of the following story, namely, some people's inclination toward sadomasochism: "I suppose, it's, er, they're even sort of, a degree of sadomasochism, that some people actually like being beaten up." The topic is introduced very cautiously through the use of the hedge "sort of" and the expanded noun phrase "a degree of," which decreases the strength of the claim that domestic violence might be attributed to sadomasochistic tendencies. Line 2 presents the protagonist of the story, "a patient," whose actions are further specified in line 3: "and she, I mean she used to come in and reg——, regale us with the, the most bizarre and, er, tales of terrible sadomastics, masochistic stuff." The verb phrase "used to" indicates a recurring pattern of this incident in the past that is reinforced by the modal auxiliary "would" in line 6 ("she'd sit there"). The implication is that this patient came regularly and thus became memorable. The other memorable feature about her was that she told "tales." By choosing this lexical item instead of the less marked "stories" or even "accounts," the GP indirectly implies that his patient's stories were so extraordinary that they almost bordered on the realm of the fantastic. This is underlined by the attributive adjective "bizarre," which is intensified through the superlative formed with "most."

   The patient's stories stood out in that they dealt with "terrible sadomasochistic stuff." The judgmental adjective "terrible" clearly gives away the doctor's disapproval of the woman's sexual practices. It is also interesting that a slip of the tongue makes the GP say "sadomastics" first before he immediately corrects himself. This might indicate the GP's excitement or embarrassment at a point where he mentions to the interviewer something "unspeakable" from the point of view of mainstream moral standards. The GP's verb choice implies that the whole incident is evaluated as being funny in retrospect. The woman "regaled" staff members with her stories. The humorous side of the story is emphasized by the GP's laughter in line 10. Laughter might indicate the GP's embarrassment about the story he relates or it might show that he finds the woman's conduct bizarre and impossible to comprehend. Another explanation for "black humor" in medical practice could be that it offers doctors a way of remaining "clinical" and of not getting too involved in difficult issues. As another male GP commented:

> 1. You just can't take it home with you. You've got to learn not to get involved in that sense. You know, you need to give them the time and the ear that's necessary but you can't take it on, take it even personal. Or you're going nuts. . . . That's why medical humor is very black. . . . I think that's, that's the reason or one of the reasons for that and why some people cannae understand it. We're a weird bunch. We are, because I think there is a one-way, a viewing of these sorts of major problems that is subtly humorous. You could see it as sick, you know [laughs]. And that's how we cope, that's how we deal with it.

While humor seems necessary as a means of psychological and emotional "self-defense," as it were, it can perhaps also be detrimental if patients' experiences are downplayed and ridiculed and not taken seriously anymore.

Despite the "terrible" sadomasochistic practices, the patient in this story stayed with her husband for a lengthy period, "ten years," which is made explicit and is also evaluated as incomprehensible behavior through the contrastive connector "but": "but she stayed with her husband for ten years, you know" (line 4). In line 5 the patient's behavior is then labeled as pathological through the adjective "schizoid": "it was, um, you know, it, it was, it was almost sort of schizoid." In a sense the GP reconstructs his patient as deviant and abnormal. This discursive strategy is toned down, however, by the two preceding hedges, "almost" and "sort of," which can be regarded as indirect disclaimers to the GP's evaluation. Lines 6 to 10 form the core of the whole story because the GP reenacts a scene as it occurred between himself and this patient: "she'd sit there and say, 'He's doing this, that, and the other,' you know, '[took] me and beat me up' and 'Why don't you leave?' 'Oh, I can't leave!' [laughs], you know." By using dialogue the GP dramatizes the encounter for the listener. As Tannen points out, giving "voice to the speech of people who are depicted as taking part in events . . . creates a play peopled by characters who take on life and breath" (1989:103). The purpose of such dramatizations is to interest the listener and to create involvement.

The GP's minidrama is marked by extremely short clauses and by ellipsis. Thus, in line 7 the verb phrase is shortened from "she would say" to just "say," and in lines 8 to 10 the *verba dicendi* introducing the reported speech are left out completely. The use of ellipsis heightens the dramatic effect of this scene because the patient's and the doctor's turns at talk are immediately juxtaposed, and thus the whole scene comes to life in front of the listener. The reported speech is not really "reported" but rather "constructed," as Tannen argues, since the words are not likely to be exactly those of the speakers at the time. When the GP rephrases his patient's accounts as "He's doing this, that, and the other," for example, he already summarizes her various stories in an unspecified manner. The point of replaying the scene rather than just telling the listener about it is to present a scene that approximately captures the gist of what actually took place on several occasions. Ultimately, the GP tries to convey to the interviewer what exactly was so "funny" about these encounters, namely, the woman's bizarre stories and her strange behavior.

As I mentioned above, this story was related spontaneously during a discussion of possible reasons for domestic violence. The fact that the GP chose this extremely unusual case as an example underlines my assumption that primarily those cases become part of GPs' memorized stock of "storied knowledge" that are uncommon, extraordinary, or at least in some way "different" from standard cases. Standard cases may be stored more generally as scripts (see chapter 4), but they do not seem to be labeled and indexed as "special" narratives for retrieval in storytelling situations. We might infer from this that circumstances accompanying "normal" or more common cases are not remembered as well as unusual circumstances, which may ultimately lead to GPs' lack of sensitivity to less obvious signs of abuse presented by a patient during the consultation. At the same time there is a danger of setting up rather unusual cases as standard frames of reference and to reinforce cultural myths rather than to tackle the reality many women have to face.

Unusual Cases and the Mechanisms of Stereotyping

Many of the GPs' narratives present stereotypical rather than extraordinary cases. Thus, the narratives regularly suggested alcohol and drug abuse, a deprived social background, and a family history of domestic violence over generations as the main reasons for domestic violence, as I discussed in chapter 6.

Nevertheless, even these stories can be classified as "unusual," since they portray violent relationships only partially and leave out the fact that violence occurs in supposedly "normal" families as well. In my discussion of the construction of "deviance" above I already pointed out that some GPs expressed their surprise about the fact that they occasionally encountered domestic violence in seemingly "decent" patients. Stereotypes can be defined as "cognitive preconceptions" (LaFrance and Hahn 1994). As LaFrance and Hahn point out, stereotypes occur "when target individuals are classified by others as having something in common because they are perceived to be members of a particular group. Stereotypes are often associated with salient physical characteristics such as ethnicity, age, physical attractiveness, and of course, gender" (1994:352). At the same time, stereotypes are often used as explanatory frameworks for our understanding of social groups, as I discussed in chapter 1: "The outcome of the process of stereotype formation is the derivation of knowledge about categories that serves to explain similarities and differences on relevant dimensions at that time in ways which are shared. We can put it no more succinctly than to say: we form stereotypes to explain aspects of and relations between social groups" (McGarty, Spears, and Yzerbyt 2002:198–99). Interestingly enough, research in cognitive psychology has shown that "memory for infrequent events is actually poorer than memory for frequent events" (Spears 2002:136). If stereotype formation is partially based on observed facts and people's perceptions of reality, this would suggest that GPs are more aware of stereotypical or extraordinary cases. The following account given by an early-middle-aged female GP in a hospital-based health center illustrates the mechanism of stereotyping with regard to victims of domestic violence as it can be found in most of the interviews:

> 2. Um, so, a lot of times, it's, you may see someone with bruises but it's actually **not till months after that it comes out** that actually the cause of that was, er, you know, their partner. Or the other thing is it's just taken as being part of their everyday, you know, that they, they'll always explain how, or **disguise** things like their, **their partner's taking them by the neck and pinning them up against the wall and things** but that's part of, you know, they wouldn't consider leaving them, that's **just part of the relationship** and how it's, it's always

been and when you ch———, you know, challenge them about that, whether they want to do anything about that, **it's just never crossed their mind** because, often they come from an **abusive family background** as well. This is **what they're in a way used to.** Um, I mean, I haven't seen a great deal of bad bruising and things, it's been, it's been more things that have been reported afterwards or, you know, maybe when they've left the relationship they're able to, er, explore it more because it obviously has legacies if they go into another relationship as well about how they feel about their new partner, too, but, I mean, I certainly had some with, you know, fairly significant, um, bruisings as well. **Some of them because it's the drug scene,** you know, if, if **their partner's actually their pimp as well** then, you know, there's, there's obviously even more implications there if, if there's a, a problem with **the kind of business side of things** as well. We've got **a few ladies who, who are kind of professional prostitutes,** if you like, and that can become a problem, too.

This GP starts her account of her experiences with a similar thematic line to that drawn in narrative 32, namely, that instances of domestic violence are often revealed only after awhile. As I discussed in chapter 4, this can be regarded as one type of "standard scenario." The violent episode depicted ("their partner's taking them by the neck and pinning them up against the wall and things"), however, is more reminiscent of the dramatized action presented in narrative 15, where the GP also spoke about the victim as being "pinned to the wall." Another interesting point to note here is again the attribution of agency to the women. Women find explanations for their partner's violence and "disguise" what is really happening, thereby assuming an active part in their victimization. On the other hand, they remain inactive and stay in a violent relationship partly because "it's never crossed their mind" to leave. This statement almost portrays women victims as lacking judgment and common sense, and, as I argued in previous chapters, it neglects other important factors such as financial or emotional dependence and fear influencing women's decision to stay. An "abusive family background" is offered as one explanation, which is as stereotypical as the connection between violence and drug abuse pointed out: "Some of them because it's the drug scene, you know."

Evaluating the Severity of Domestic Violence Cases

This GP indirectly also distinguishes between two types of domestic violence cases, namely, those with or without "significant bruisings." The cases where the GP did not see any "bad bruisings" are said to be "reported afterwards," and they are contrasted with some "fairly significant" bruisings: "I mean, I certainly had some with, you know, fairly significant, um, bruisings as well." Interestingly enough, the GP's reference to significant cases is immediately followed by scenarios with rather extraordinary circumstances. Thus, the GP alludes to the drug scene and to the milieu of prostitutes and their pimps, and she establishes a causal relationship between these backgrounds and violence by using the logical connector "because." Once again, the myth that violence is related to social background is reinforced. Although this account is not, strictly speaking, a narrative, as it does not depict a particular case, the GP nonetheless obeys Labov's rule of the "most reportable event." The fact that uncommon, extraordinary cases are indirectly associated with significance and memorability obviously raises problems for the way doctors might deal with domestic violence cases.

Domestic abuse only seems to be considered a "real" problem if the case is severe or if there is a sensational outcome. This underpins the following findings by Lamb concerning the construction of images of victims:

> The expectation that an abuse victim will develop symptoms is clear. It is also clear that victims' suffering must be long and severe, or else their victimization is trivial and does not "count." This expectation is endorsed, ironically, both by victim advocates who cannot believe that someone's abuse is not the central meaning-making incident in their lives and by backlash authors who do not count minor abusive experiences as "real" abuse, calling victims "whiners" for so labeling these experiences. For abuse to count, the suffering can never go away. (1999:113)

In other words, there is a tendency for people to distinguish degrees of salience of domestic violence cases. In the context of medical care this practice of compartmentalizing victims into "severe" or "less severe" cases can have far-reaching consequences if doctors adjust their own help resources depending on whether they think a woman "really needs" and "deserves" help or not.

Stereotyped Taboos and Their Impact on Talk-in-Interaction

Another striking linguistic feature in the excerpt above, especially toward the end, is the frequent use of hedges. Hedges are commonly used by speakers to avoid loss of face and to fulfill the face wants of the interlocutor (Brown and Levinson 1987). They typically qualify and tone down statements "in order to reduce the riskiness of what one says" (Wales 2001:185). In other words, speakers try not to offend their interlocutors by what they say. At the same time, hedges are often an indication of reluctance to talk openly about a certain topic. In the extract above the GP's use of hedges increases when she starts to talk about the "significant bruisings" and the whole drug and prostitution scene. Apart from the frequent discourse markers "I mean," "you know," and "um," the GP repeats the connectors "if" and "who," the indexical determiner "there's," and the indefinite article "a." More important, the GP uses the hedges "a kind of" twice in connection with the noun phrases "business side of things" and "professional prostitutes." This reveals the GP's reluctance to speak about the topic of prostitution and may be attributed to her wish not to offend the interviewer or to her embarrassment about this topic, which is generally regarded as morally despicable in our society because it involves associations of deviant sexuality, crime, improper behavior, indecency, and so on. The GP's sense of embarrassment is also revealed by the phrase "if you like" ("We've got a few ladies who, who are kind of professional prostitutes, if you like"), which shows that the GP is uncertain about the wording of what she wants to say. The phrase implies that the GP signals to the interviewer that the lexical items chosen in this context are perhaps not ideal, but, at the same time, the GP tries to reassure herself of the interviewer's approval of her word choice. This passage demonstrates that the level of self-monitoring in speech can be high, especially if GPs talk about issues that they are presumably not familiar with firsthand and that they may consider inappropriate in a formal context like the interview or an unsuitable topic to discuss with a young, female researcher.

Silence, Hedges, and Euphemisms:
Discursive Evasions of a Taboo Topic

Since domestic violence is generally still considered a family or private issue (although, in fact, the repercussions and resulting costs affect everyone [Schornstein 1997:26]), people often treat the problem as taboo and find it difficult to talk about it. This could also be felt in the interviews when hedges and pauses indicated reluctance on the part of the doctor to express violent acts directly and openly, for example. Pauses are often deployed in narratives to create suspense. As Auer, Couper-Kuhlen, and Müller point out, the "story is initiated and then saliently interrupted at a turning point where crucial further events can be expected. . . . Breaking up a locally established isochronous rhythmic progression at the 'point of incidence' . . . is an effective synaesthetic linguistic means to contextualize this suspense-creating strategy" (1999:180). In the following narrative related by an older female GP pause and hedging underline the theme of secrecy mentioned in the story and even enact it on the discourse level of the narrative.

Narrative 8

1. there's a, a patient I've got at the moment
2. and I think her husband mistreats her.
3. and, hem, um, the husband tends to come with the wife
4. and of course she's not going to say that she's [pause],
5. so, it may be even more hidden in an ethnic grouping than it is in the Eu——, er, Western grouping. Yeah.

Narrative 8 is not typical of an oral narrative in the Labovian sense, as it employs present tense rather than the more common past tense. Simple present, which is normally used to indicate a general state, habitual action, or sometimes instantaneous action (Quirk et al. 1985:179–80), shows, on the one hand, a clear reference to the present time (also expressed in the temporal adverbial phrase "at the moment" in line 1) and, on the other hand, the habitual aspect of the patient's visits in company of her husband: "the husband *tends* to come with the wife" (line 3, my emphasis). The simple present in line 5, by contrast, expresses a general state of affairs as perceived by the GP. The statement, however, is modified by the modal auxiliary "may" as a not entirely certain possibility assumed by the GP: "it may be even more hidden in an ethnic grouping" (line 5). In other words, instead of depicting a particular instance of a consultation with this patient, the doctor refers to this case in more general terms, thus also setting it up as an example of the occurrence of domestic violence in ethnic groups.

What is significant in this setting is the secrecy with which abuse is associated, as can be seen in the adjectival participle "hidden" (line 5). Interestingly enough, however, not only is this secrecy mentioned in the text, but the narrative itself epitomizes secrecy. Thus, for example, the GP uses euphemism to describe violence: "I think her husband mistreats her" (line 2). Rather than using verbs such as "abuse," "beat," and so on, the GP falls back on a more neutral term that does not necessarily include physical violence and thus blurs the concept. The statement therefore becomes more tentative. This is reinforced by the "hedged performative" (Fraser 1975) "I think," which expresses uncertainty about whether violence is really at stake in this couple.[1] The interjections "hem" and "um" in line 3 create a short discursive pause that I interpret as showing the GP's reluctance to talk about this case or her attempt to find appropriate words to formulate the narrative. Either way, a sense of embarrassment is conveyed in this somewhat evasive presentation, and this becomes particularly obvious in the lengthy pause in line 4, where the GP simply breaks off the sentence: "and of course she's not going to say that she's [pause]." Silence exactly coincides with the point of the narrative that deals with the patient's silence. On the one hand, the narrative's *discourse* thus enacts and replicates the contents of the *story*; on the other hand, it demonstrates that silence is imposed not only on the victim's language but also on that of the responsible GP. As much as the patient "hides" her problem from the doctor, the GP also holds back an explicit verbal expression of her suspicion in the interview. In a sense, narrative 8 thus demonstrates how potential service providers might indirectly collude with the secrecy of victims and thus help perpetuate domestic violence rather than challenge it. Mutual embarrassment between doctor and patient about a taboo topic such as domestic violence may thus lead to the same paradox that Trinch observed for the discussion of rape in legal advice settings: "Ironically, it may be that the nearly universal sociocultural repugnance against this condemned act is precisely what contributes to the seeming hesitation of victims to come forward for help, as service providers too seem to prefer to hear about other, perhaps culturally less offensive or at least conversationally less sensitive, acts of violence" (2001b:601). Applied to the context of domestic violence in general practice, a tendency for euphemism and silence in GPs' narrative practices can be detrimental, as it might suggest to women that their "personal" problems are not desirable topics in a consultation, which in turn may lead to a general hush-up of domestic abuse.

Female-on-Male Violence

Most of the narratives presented so far are unusual because they display a high degree of violence or because the actors in these stories are to some extent "deviant" in terms of general moral standards. Narrative 15 stands out, for example, because the perpetrator of the violence is a female student. Although violence is still mainly perpetrated by men on women (Williamson 2000:6), nine of the male GPs and seven of the female GPs mentioned female-on-male violence at some point in the interview, and a few doctors (significantly enough, men) elaborated on such cases in their practices. Most of the time female-on-male violence was alluded to only in passing. The following examples illustrate this. Note that the statements presented in (3) were given by male doctors and the ones in (4) by female doctors.

3. a. Eventually they'll come. And **only this year, for the first time I've seen two men.**

b. I don't feel uncomfortable discussing these things with my patients. **I also had one man who was abused, by the way.**

c. I think we mostly see, um, domestic violence in terms of, er, um, man on female. **It does happen the other way round as well** but the men don't come and tell us about it so much.

d. I think there's a hidden, huge hidden, you know, mass of it that no one comes forward and I've never known of a male being assaulted **but I know that men do get assaulted by their wives.**

e. And **the last person I had in who'd been complaining of being hit was actually a man** who was complaining that his girlfriend had been beating him up. So . . . [**laughs**]

f. And the other one will be "My husband hit me" or "partner hit" [clears his throat] and **occasionally it's, it's the other way around where the male's been, er, assaulted.**

g. I suppose it's often difficulties in relationships or just that, um, some people are, well, well, **we know some women beat up men as**

well but it's some, some sort of way their character has been formed and that's the way they, they deal with their relationships.

4. a. You often get it maybe after the couple have separated and you're seeing the wife with depression. Um, **there's also the husband some-times that gets beaten up but that's not so common** [laughs].

b. I think it is. Sort of just power, **but then of course women beat up men.**

c. There's no rhyme nor reason to it. **Occasionally you come across women who are abusing their husbands but it's more often the other way round, definitely, yeah.**

d. Um, there's also the other sort of issue of confidentiality, I mean, the abuser, **whether it be the husband that's the abuser or the wife that's the abuser,** they're often patients of me as well.

e. I can't imagine why any man would want to, you know, presum-ing it's a man hitting a woman **although obviously it can be other ways round** but, you know, it's just very cowardly.

f. I don't think they think consciously "Right, I'm the one to take that power over you," um, it just happens. Um, I mean I'm sure, sure **that might happen the other way round as well but it's not that common, I don't think.**

Although these allusions to female-on-male violence are, on the whole, fairly similar, one can notice a few differences between the men's and the women's responses. First of all, as already mentioned, male GPs referred more often to particular cases they had come across in their practice work ("only this year, for the first time I've seen two men" [3a]; "I also had one man who was abused" [3b]; "the last person I had in who'd been complaining of being hit was actu-ally a man" [3e]), while the women's statements are always formulated in gen-eral terms. A lot of the GPs mentioned female-on-male violence while they were discussing reasons for domestic violence, but, in addition to that, female GPs brought it up in the context of power relations, as in (4b) and (4f): "Sort of just power," "I don't think they think consciously 'Right, I'm the one to take that power over you.'" Interestingly enough, female-on-male violence is introduced in these examples as a counterargument against the feminist proposition I suggested in the interview that violence is possibly related to men's power and dominance in our patriarchal society. Female GPs stated more regularly that female-on-male violence was rare compared to male-on-female violence, while male GPs sometimes took the opportunity to make an ironical comment or to present a particular case in a joking manner. Laughter indicated GPs' amusement about the idea of female-on-male violence, and it may be interpreted as GPs' response to something that contradicts their expectations of manhood and virility. Only one female GP laughed ("Um, there's also the husband sometimes that gets beaten up but that's not so common [laughs]" [4a]) but, significantly, she was nearing retirement, and we might assume that her ideas of manhood were relatively conservative, inducing her to find the idea of a battered man "funny." Another explanation might be that this GP felt embarrassed about the issue and laughed to cover up her feeling. One middle-aged male GP was amused by the fact that "one guy has got a bigger beating-up than many women I have come across," and another male GP commented, laughing, "I mean if I was with a wife like this, it's absolutely terrible." As I argued above, humor in these instances might also point toward the ways in which GPs try to deal with difficult and professionally taxing situations.

Female-on-Male Violence and the Evocation of Gender Stereotypes

The response in (3g) is interesting as it demonstrates once again how male GPs sometimes presented violence as more deviant and as a result of a pathological character trait if it was perpetrated by a woman: "I suppose it's often difficulties in relationships or just that, um, some people are, well, well, we know some women beat up men as well but it's some, some sort of way their character has been formed and that's the way they, they deal with their relationships." The GP talks first about reasons for domestic violence in general, focusing on "difficulties in relationships." By using this vague noun phrase the GP implicitly attributes the cause of violence equally to both partners, as it does not become clear who is responsible for the difficulties. As soon as the GP mentions female-on-male violence, however, the explanation for it is a lot more clearly defined: it is "some sort of way their [i.e., the women's] character has been formed." In other words, both in male-on-female as in female-on-male violence the cause is more likely to be attributed to the woman, or, as Bograd (1987:73) puts it, women are "defined as the locus of the problem." Consider the following comment made by a late-middle-aged male GP:

> 5. There are a few men that I am aware of, of, er, being subject to bat-tering from their spouses. But they don't come forward so often. You know, quite vicious attacks sometimes, knives, pots and pans and, premenstrual tension has been [blamed a great deal for this].

Women's violence is depicted and, at the same time, evaluated in negative terms, as "quite vicious attacks." The adjective "vicious" implies women's evil inten-tions, that is, the cause of violence is clearly ascribed to the female perpetra-tor. This contrasts with other depictions of "standard" violence cases where agency and causation are often blurred, as I discussed above. The weapons this GP mentions—"knives, pots and pans"—evoke the stereotypical, traditional scenario of "woman in the house and kitchen." This cliché is supplemented by another common prejudice often cited to account for women's "irrational" be-havior, namely, "premenstrual tension." Again, violence in these rather excep-tional cases is depicted as something inherent in females. Interestingly enough, in a first round of pilot interviews PMS was used by a male GP as an explana-tion for male-on-female violence in the sense that men "tend to react" to their wives' irrational behavior instead of "just walking away." This type of gender-related explanation underlines Bograd's assumption that doctors' approaches to battered women are largely based on "prevailing male-defined cultural myths about women" (1987:69). There is possibly a gender issue underlying doctor-patient interaction with regard to domestic violence if the GP is a man, as male GPs might find it more difficult to fully empathize with their female patients. On the other hand, large parts of the GPs' responses are very similar in tone and topic, which indicates that the problem might be related to other factors such as divergent life experiences and backgrounds, as I argued above.

Narrative Gaps and the Evaluation of Female-on-Male Violence
Sometimes what people do *not* talk about can be equally revealing as what they *do* talk about in an interview. One male GP nearing retirement, for example,

when asked about his experiences and whether there was a case he remembered in particular, did *not* relate a narrative about male-on-female violence, the more common form of domestic abuse, but instead elaborated a narrative about a man who was abused by his wife:

Narrative 14

J: Yeah. Um, is there any case that's particularly vivid in your memory, anything that was . . .

1. I think possibly, er, the one and only time I've ever come across a, um, an abused man.
2. Because I'd read about them
3. but it took me completely by surprise when I actually met one
4. because he was a big-bellied chap who actually ran away from Dundee
5. and allegedly a very small, er, wife who did, er, exhibit, er, violence towards him.
6. And again I couldn't understand, er,
7. [I'll] never be able to understand why [you have to use] violence in a relationship
8. but I couldn't understand why he accepted it for so long
9. but again, there was, he was a chap on the road.
10. I didn't see him for very long,
11. I never established the truth of the situation.

Analysis of Narrative 14

Narrative cohesion is established through a number of repetitions and parallel structures here. Thus, lines 4 and 5 ("a big-bellied chap who," "a very small wife who") and lines 7 and 8 ("I'll never be able to understand why," "I couldn't understand why") are marked by syntactic parallelisms, and among the repetitions the verb "understand" stands out because it appears in three consecutive clauses in lines 6, 7, and 8: "And again I couldn't understand, er, I'll never be able to understand why you have to use violence in a relationship but I couldn't understand why he accepted it for so long." This repetition emphasizes the focal point of the GP's evaluation, namely, the fact that he can understand neither people's reasons for violence in general nor the patient's reason for accepting violence. The narrative starts with the orientation part: "I think possibly, er, the one and only time I've ever come across a, um, an abused man." In this orientation the narrator sets up a temporal framework by stressing the fact that the incident related in the following story occurred only once in the past: it was the "one and only time" that the GP "ever" saw an abused man. The phrasal verb "come across" with its underlying *path metaphor* (Lakoff and Johnson 1980), which can be seen in the use of the spatial preposition "across," implies that the encounter with an abused man was experienced as something unexpected and unforeseen and thus also as something unusual. The mental image that is conjured up is one of the GP "stumbling" over this peculiar case in his hitherto "smooth" path of practice encounters with domestic violence cases. It "took" the GP "completely by surprise" when he "actually met" an abused man (line 3). The adverb "actually" emphasizes the real-life experience in contrast to what the GP had "read about them" (line 2). The whole encounter is presented like a scientist's first encounter with a rare disease or a less well researched species, which is reinforced by the collective third-person plural pronoun "them" in line 2 and the numeral "one" in line 3: "Because I'd read about them but it took me completely by surprise when I actually met one." The GP thus indirectly sets up a category of people who could be classified as "abused men," and this category is depicted as nonstandard or outside the norm. By conveying the rarity of such occurrences the GP justifies his telling of this story. He signals to the interviewer that the narrative contains a "reportable event" and that it is therefore worth telling.

The protagonists in this story are described in contrastive terms in lines 4 and 5. While the man is colloquially depicted as "a big-bellied chap," his wife is only "very small," which makes it even more remarkable, in the GP's view, that the man should have suffered abuse from his partner. The focus on people's physical size is reminiscent of narrative 15, where the GP also emphasized the size of the female perpetrator. This points toward a notion of violence as being correlated with mere physical strength and thus reveals again a common cliché about the issue. What strikes us as unusual in the GP's depiction of the violent action is the formality of the verb "exhibit" ("allegedly a very small, er, wife who did, er, exhibit, er, violence towards him" [line 5]), which stands in stark contrast to the previously colloquial tone and also diminishes linguistically the strength of the violent act, as it remains neutral and distanced. This discursive contrast highlights the discrepancy between doctors as a professional or expert group and as a folk group that also uses folk language.

The fact that the referential meaning of the verb "exhibit" as such does not entail violence underlines a "clinical" register that incorporates the discursive strategy of disassociation. The reason for this strategy can be found in the GP's doubtful attitude, which is expressed in the adverb "allegedly" and in the last evaluative statement in line 11: "I never established the truth of the situation." The GP implicitly conveys his uncertainty about the truth condition of this case, and the case is thus presented as a story with an open ending. The reason for this is that the GP "didn't see" the patient for a long time, as he "was a chap on the road" (line 9). This causal relationship can be established if we interpret lines 9 to 11 ("but again, there was, he was a chap on the road. I didn't see him for very long, I never established the truth of the situation") as a logical sequence, with the cause provided in line 9, followed by its consequence and the overall implication of this connection. Does the GP link the patient's lifestyle with the occurrence of violence and thus reinforce the cultural myth that violence is related to social class? Or does he imply a relationship between the man's lifestyle and his acceptance of violence, thereby drawing upon the stereotype of the "deviant other"? Or is the man's life "on the road" simply mentioned to explain the fact that the GP was unable to find out the truth, since the patient did not come regularly?

At any rate, this narrative contains the same discursive strategies and themes that can be found in other narratives in my sample as well, for example, the GP's surprise and initial incredulity, stereotyping in terms of physical size and social background, and, finally, the GP's lack of understanding in view of a violent relationship. The clause in line 7 ("I'll never be able to understand"), which moves temporally outside the story time through its future tense marker, states not only in a negative but also in a categorical tone that the GP simply cannot understand the use of violence in a relationship. As I mentioned above, this is a view a great number of the GPs in my sample expressed in the interviews but mostly in terms of the more common male-on-female violence. It is interesting that this GP related a narrative in the same fashion as most of the other GPs related "normal" cases of male-on-female violence, albeit unusual in other respects, as I discussed above. The fact that this particular narrative was selected in the context of the interview indicates that the case depicted by this GP must have been labeled and stocked as noteworthy and reportable, whereas the more common cases of male-on-female violence do not seem to feature prominently in the GP's memory or are at least not considered interesting enough to be related in a storytelling situation. In other words, it is once again the extraordinary that receives attention by means of narrative evaluation, while less conspicuous cases, which probably reflect better the everyday reality women experience, are excluded from the GP's "storied knowledge."

Female-on-Male Violence and GPs' Narrative Knowledge

Yet again, the story the GP remembered vividly was one that contains some extraordinary element. It looks as though doctors' perceptions of domestic violence and of the circumstances surrounding it are based on extraordinary, unusual, or stereotypical cases they remember and reproduce in their narratives, while other realities (e.g., violence in "normal" middle-class families or more hidden forms of violence such as psychological and verbal abuse) may be present as basic knowledge schemata but do not pertain to the more vivid and particularized narrative knowledge base and thus to the narrative reality created in GPs' minds. The mentioning of female-on-male violence by most of the GPs is a striking example. Although this is in fact a rare scenario compared to the more common cases of male-on-female violence, male GPs in particular commented, sometimes in a joking manner, on cases they had had, or they elaborated on such cases in narratives. These narratives are in line with other narratives related in the interviews, as they also contain an unusual element. For example, violence related to alcohol comes to be regarded as a "standard" scene or background for domestic violence, while in reality research has shown that there is no inherent causal relationship between alcohol abuse and violent behavior and that instead men's violent behavior can be attributed to their attitudes toward women in general (Johnson 2001).

If these are the kinds of stories that doctors stock and remember in detail, while less obvious or "insignificant" cases are only memorized as general scripts, as we saw in chapter 4, this has far-reaching implications for GPs' practice work. GPs' knowledge may thus, in the worst case, lack necessary information on indirect signs of abuse and on the complexities of relationships in which domestic violence occurs as well as the complex psychological processes that underlie both victims' and perpetrators' actions and behavior. My data pose a paradox in this respect: while the GPs displayed at least theoretical knowledge about "hidden signs" of abuse, their particularized narratives of actual experiences focus more on extraordinary cases. Moreover, as I outlined in chapter 3, GPs frequently miss cases. The explanation I propose here against the background of the cognitive approaches to narrative mentioned above is that GPs perhaps do not stock less dramatic cases in their memories and consequently are less sensitized to more hidden signs of abuse.

Ironically, there is, then, a mismatch between doctors' "experiential" knowledge about a problem that does not fit the biomedical model and the factual reality they encounter but perhaps do not fully recognize in their daily practice work. This lack of adequate narrative knowledge of a psychosocial problem can lead to other problems, including misdiagnoses and subsequent wrong treatment such as the prescription of drugs. As Williamson's interviews with victims of domestic violence revealed, women are often prescribed drugs paradoxically in situations when such drugs can potentially do more harm than good. Drugs "can be damaging to a woman's sense of safety, place her in a position where she can act out para-suicidal tendencies, and reinforce a lack of control within the help-seeking process" (Williamson 2000:58). All this points toward special requirements as far as medical training is concerned. I will turn to this question in my final chapter.

9. Conclusion

Narrative research has seen an incredible proliferation over the last four decades, and the term *narrative* seems to be almost a buzzword in a great number of disciplines now. It is perhaps not surprising, then, that narrative research has also called forth critics who consider current interests in narrative a passing fashion. I hope that I have managed to dissipate some of the skepticism some readers may initially have felt and that my book has shown the importance of narrative research for the investigation of social problems such as domestic violence. Let me briefly address again some of the critical observations generally held against narrative before I summarize the findings of my study.

One point of criticism is that narrative is perhaps not as universal a feature as is often claimed, that it is highly dependent on cultural context, and that it constitutes only a small part of a whole gamut of verbal and nonverbal forms of interaction. Thus, it is important to consider the immediate context out of which narratives emerge and to analyze the narratives within larger sociocultural frameworks, especially where sociocultural problems such as domestic violence are at stake. This is a valid argument that needs to be taken into account in any research set within the narrative paradigm and to which I have given sufficient attention in this book. It is true that human interaction is also performative, that is, it is based on gestures, glances, body language, and other nonlinguistic signals, and ideally some of this should also be considered in narrative research. However, people negotiate what they think and feel and know through language, and it is mainly these *discursive* negotiations that formed the data for my narrative-analytic approach. Narratives lend themselves as research material as they accommodate both sociocultural discourse, which "speaks through" individuals, as it were, as well as individual people's perspectives. Narratives facilitate both an intellectual and emotional sharing of ideas and of human experience, a sharing that, as a number of philosophers contend, lies outside of hardcore natural science and cannot be fully grasped by "scientific method" alone. And, as I demonstrated in this study, sometimes it is exactly the discrepancy between scientific and narrative paradigms that can lead to the aggravation of social problems such as domestic violence.

Another point of criticism often raised against narrative research is that it conflates an analytical framework with the data it investigates. As with other qualitative research methods, it is probably true that one cannot make a clear-cut distinction between the data one wishes to analyze and the tools one uses for analyzing them. Thus, narratives are commonly elicited by means of "narrative interviews," for example. This need not be a flaw, however. In fact, one of the great strengths of narrative research, I would argue, is that it enables one to transform the research object in the very process of researching it. Thus, by trying to understand what the narrative mechanisms underlying GPS' narratives about domestic violence cases are and by trying to do this through narrative interviews, I became more aware of my own and other people's narrative practices and I hope also raised awareness in the GPS. One GP commented at the end of the interview: "Um, and perhaps it's like all these other things, like depression or all that, we should, we should have our feelers out a bit more just to see if we could pick it up. Um, I'm certainly more aware of it having spoken about it today, you know, next time I'll probably be asking everybody if they [laughs], um." As Eastern philosophies have it, the way is already the goal, the method the result. On this note let me summarize the results of my study in this concluding chapter.

The GPS' Narratives Revisited

The twenty interviews yield very interesting and diverse results. Nevertheless, some patterns can be found that mark many of the interviews and thus contribute to a sense of similarity and overlap. In chapter 2 I hypothesize that, if it was possible to find common features in the GPS' narratives or even a common narrative pattern, we should also be able to identify a linguistic "community of practice" (Eckert and McConnell-Ginet 1992), in this case, that of general practitioners. It would be presumptuous to claim that there is one common narrative that can be filtered out of all the GPS' responses because individual narratives in the sample do in fact provide somewhat different perspectives. However, it is not exaggerated to say that certain patterns emerge from the GPS' narrative discourses that point in the direction of some sort of discursive community of practice with specific "members' resources" (Fairclough 1989, 2001) and an "institutional memory" (Linde 1999; Trinch 2001b). This community seems to be largely informed by knowledge about domestic violence that draws upon the biomedical model, on the one hand, and common cultural myths and stereotypes concerning the problem, on the other. Thus, the most frequently quoted reasons for domestic violence in the GPs' narratives are alcohol or drug abuse; a deprived social background and a family history of violence; lack of education that is often combined with a lack of communication skills; and relationship problems. Less frequently, GPs mentioned reasons from the perpetrator's perspective, including aggressiveness and jealousy in the male partner; male dominance in general; PMS; the fact that many men nowadays feel threatened by women's growing independence; obsessive affection; and the biological "fact" that men are stronger and bigger than women and "therefore" more prone to violent behavior. Interestingly enough, the reasons from the male perspective were invariably only offered if I explicitly asked about possible reasons or if I introduced "male power" as a prompt for further discussions.

Although the GPs in my sample generally acknowledged that, according to research findings, domestic violence occurred across cultures, social classes, and age groups, most GPs re-created stereotypical backgrounds of violence in their narratives, for example, by delineating the "Saturday night ritual" when the husband goes out "on a bender" or "gets pissed" and then beats up his wife. Interestingly enough, these narratives are often very lively because scenes are linguistically reenacted by the GPs through the use of colloquial expressions and "constructed dialogue" (Tannen 1989), that is, the narrator's "reconstruction" of direct speech. In a similar fashion the GPs' narratives mostly depict not only stereotypical scenes of violence but cases of violence that were in some way extraordinary and "reportable" in Labov's (1972a) sense.

Explanations such as socialization, deprivation, and alcohol or even biological explanations regarding size, male and female social behavior, and so on are problematic, as they deflect responsibility away from the perpetrator and delegate it to external social or biological forces. Put another way, violence is almost presented as inevitable, as something that happens because of x, y, and z rather than because men do it purposefully in order to gain or keep control and to exert power or because present-day society still condones male dominance and thus indirectly legitimizes violence. By using such explanatory frameworks in their narratives GPs indirectly reinforce current "excuses" and "justifications" frequently used by batterers themselves (Ptacek 1990) and thus perpetuate the victimization of women on the institutional level of general practice.

At the same time, explanatory frameworks that relegate domestic violence to the social realm also offer a justification for doctors to deny agency to themselves. One line of reasoning that a number of GPs in my sample put forward was that domestic violence is primarily a social problem with mainly social origins, and therefore doctors' role in this context is limited. Many of the GPs stated that "there is not very much we can do about it." This attitude also seems to be mainly informed by the biomedical model, in which the doctors' role is restricted to treating illness, and it also leads to GPs' sense of inadequacy and powerlessness, which is often conveyed in metaphors such as the "tip of the iceberg" and the "can of worms" that express GPs' anxiety about dealing with domestic violence. The spatiotemporal language the GPs used to depict domestic violence revealed the problem as something that is "hidden," "low on the ground," or even "underground," hence, both threatening and difficult to detect. The reasons that GPs identified for their feeling of powerlessness as well as the fact that they might miss cases were mainly lack of time, training, and adequate resources or knowledge about resources.

Whether these are simply valid reasons or partly also excuses for inaction is very difficult to determine. At any rate, such arguments perpetuate the low status of domestic violence in general practice and thus GPs' passivity rather than encourage new perspectives and a readiness for change. The "institutional memory" created through the GPs' narratives thus ultimately impedes a paradigm shift. In other words, we can argue that if doctors do not change their discursive practices, there can be no significant change in their "institutional memory" of domestic violence cases and consequently also no major change in doctors' work practices concerning the issue. This poses questions about GPs' training that I will address in greater detail below.

Even when domestic violence is disclosed and comes "to the surface," as it were, GPs' reactions may not be helpful or may even be counterproductive. Some of the narratives that the GPs in my sample produced indicate the stigmatization and labeling of victims of domestic violence as "deviant" or as the incomprehensible "other" not only in terms of gender but also in terms of behavior. Thus, women were occasionally pathologized as "schizoid" or as "sadomasochistic." Such narratives are problematic, since they reinforce the notion that women who suffer abuse are in some way "abnormal" or "different" from other women, and they also blur the fact that psychological problems such as depression or schizophrenia may be *results* of domestic abuse rather than reasons for it (Rosewater 1990). At the same time, these explanations reinforce and perpetuate a culture of victim blaming that can be harmful in a consultation when a woman seeks support and understanding. Instead of listening to and validating victims' stories, doctors indirectly blame women for being battered.

While such narratives certainly portray extreme cases, other discursive devices, for example, the use of generalizing noun phrases such as "fights between partners" and the redefinition of violence as "relationship problems" or "disharmony in relationships" are equally damaging, as they attribute the cause of violence to both partners or blur agency and thus again implicitly put the blame on the woman. I would argue that linguistic reconstructions of domestic violence cases such as these are even more harmful than explicit forms of victim blaming, since they are less easily uncovered and thus perpetuate victimization on a subtler level. Spence describes the creation of everyday myths as follows: "Very quickly, an official narrative is established, which feeds on the details of the more sensational accounts; these become a kind of media virus that instantly infect [*sic*] all current explanations. . . . The most popular grassroots explanation, as it gathers more and more persuasive details, rapidly assumes the form of a myth with its own power to persuade and hold its ground against all kinds of disconfirming evidence" (1998:220). Applied to the GPs' narratives, this also means that women's experiences of violence may be distorted if the women are discredited or agency is blurred. It is not least for this reason that a close linguistic analysis of the GPs' narratives has proved to be a useful methodological tool.

What is also uncovered in the GPs' narrative discourses is a sense of distance between themselves and their patients. As I argued above, this distance can be the result of divergent life experiences much in the same way as doctors and patients are separated by the "wellness-illness divide" (Donald 1998). In this sense, the GPs' discourses reveal a lack of comprehension and perhaps even ignorance about a problem the GPs may never have experienced themselves. At the same time, a kind of "comfort zone" is created that keeps unpleasant or even disturbing facts of life at a distance. As Keller (1996) points out, this mechanism functions largely unconsciously and serves the purpose of emotional self-protection. The linguistic reconstruction of abuse victims as "deviant" is only one of a number of discursive strategies in this respect. In reconstructing scenes of domestic violence against the background of social deprivation and other related circumstances a distance is created between the spheres of activity and lifestyles of doctors and their patients and thus reinforces a gap in understanding that GPs themselves admitted to.

Furthermore, the close analysis of the GPs' conceptualization of the "spacetime region" (Herman 2001) of the consultation, for example, shows that GPs view their own role as "static" and passive, while the patient moves along a vector in and out of the practice and in a way "passes by." A sense of distance clearly emerges from the GPs' spatiotemporal mappings. Thus, the journey metaphor and the path schema employed in the GPs' narratives indicate that women are allocated different paths and locations from their GPs' (they are presented as being "out there," as having to "find a way," or as being sent "on their way"), while GPs "go down the physical route" in consultations (they follow the path opened to them within the biomedical framework, which involves primarily treating physical injuries). Since the GP has only a very limited view or "gaze" (Foucault 1973; Young 1997) of the patient and her personal and private background, which is often even reduced to the "pink sheet" in front of the doctor during a consultation, it becomes extremely difficult for the GP to discover or sense underlying problems unless the patient volunteers that kind of information. GPs often stressed that they wished patients would assume a more active role in disclosing domestic abuse, while, ironically, women seem to expect their doctors to help them to speak up by asking appropriate questions (Williamson 2000). This again indicates a distance and a lack of relevant communication between doctor and patient that can stem from different reasons: first, both doctor and patient may feel constrained by the fact that domestic violence is still a taboo subject and may thus refrain from discussing it, as raising the issue might be interpreted as intrusive by the other party. Second, GPs might deliberately overlook the issue and enforce a "comfort zone" between themselves and their patients in order to maintain the "ceremonial order" (Strong 1979) of the consultation because they do not feel adequately equipped to deal with domestic violence.

Domestic violence is out of the GPs' reach not only spatially but, it seems, also cognitively in the sense that doctors' storied knowledge draws upon a limited set of explanatory narratives that, as I maintained, are informed by a restricted "medical gaze" and the same laypersons' knowledge about the problem that can be found in the media and other nonscientific sources. Thus, narratives were related where there was a fatal or at least sensational outcome or where perpetrators used a high degree of violence; where victims and perpetrators were alcoholics or drug addicts or even prostitutes and pimps; or where the woman had a sadomasochistic streak or was "schizoid" or deviant in some way or another, as I mentioned above. In the analysis I proposed two main reasons for why GPs might have chosen to relate these "unusual" narratives in the interviews: one explanation concerns cultural expectations about what a "good story" should be like; the other one is related to GPs' memorized stock of storied knowledge about domestic abuse. Thus, we can assume that GPs related unusual cases because they thought that was expected in the interview, given the fact that in our culture "good" stories must contain some element that is exciting, extraordinary, or "reportable" (Labov 1972a). At the same time, however, if we accept the argument that narratives represent and also re-create our knowledge about people, experiences, and incidents, the GPs' narratives indicate that their knowledge of domestic violence is very selective and that it is indeed informed by common cultural myths and clichés about domestic violence.

Significantly, none of the GPs in my sample mentioned the guidelines on dealing with domestic violence published by the British Medical Association (1998) or the resource manual for the medical profession that was disseminated by the Department of Health (2000) before the interviews were conducted. Instead, GPs spoke about articles they had read in the newspaper about the Zero Tolerance campaign;[1] short TV spots on the problem; media gossip about Rita Johnson, Paul Young, Paul "Gazza" Gascoigne, Sean Connery, and Mike Tyson; and the Jordache family in the British television soap opera *Brookside*. One GP mentioned a play she had seen years before that dealt with domestic violence, and another GP from the pilot interviews spoke about Roddy Doyle's novel *The Woman Who Walked into Doors* (1998) as a piece of writing that had brought domestic violence more poignantly to her attention.

What do such responses reveal with regard to GPs' narrative knowledge? First of all, these responses show that doctors are not merely professional experts but are also part of a folk group, and therefore they also draw upon "folk" discourse on domestic abuse. Moreover, the GPs' knowledge about domestic violence is "narrative," that is, it is informed by common narratives that pervade current nonacademic discourses on this topic. This kind of knowledge, however, unless it is filtered through a critical lens, might convey sensational and distorted images of victims and perpetrators of abuse and offer explanatory frameworks that are based less on "facts" of domestic violence than on simplistic stereotypes and false preconceptions (Meyers 1997). If such images and explanations are incorporated into GPS' memorized knowledge base, then there is a danger that GPS might bring this knowledge to bear on the consultation, which in turn might prove counterproductive if not harmful when a woman comes to seek help and support. In other words, if GPS reproduce sensational or at least unusual narratives about cases, they also create the realities conveyed in these narratives as a given and thus perpetuate stereotypical notions of domestic violence and images of women who suffer abuse that stigmatize as well as further victimize them. What is therefore needed, I would argue, is a paradigmatic change in doctors' narrative knowledge as well as in their narrative practices concerning psychosocial problems such as domestic violence. How this change might be brought about will be addressed in the following, final section.

Narrative Teaching Modules in the Medical Curriculum

The study presented here demonstrates in what ways narrative analysis can contribute to the uncovering and identification of a social problem such as GPS' attitudes toward domestic violence. However, the aim of this book comprises more than applying narrative expertise to the unraveling of a problem: I also wish to offer at least the beginnings of possible solutions from within the narrative framework. The question, then, is, What does the study of narrative have to offer to doctors in order for them to increase their awareness about domestic violence and to improve their medical response? The narratives elicited in the interviews clearly indicate that two major influences on GPS' conceptualizations of the problem need to be tackled: assumptions stemming from the biomedical model, on the one hand, and common cultural myths and clichés, on the other. First and foremost, however, it is imperative to bridge the gap between doctor and patient and to enhance understanding and empathy. On the one hand, GPS need to learn about women's narrative practices in the context of disclosure in order not to restrict women's stories by focusing too much on the requirements of medical record keeping and the limitations placed on doctor-patient encounters, for example. Furthermore, they ought to be able to validate women's own narratives rather than impose an institutional narrative. As Ainsworth-Vaughn has argued in her study of cancer patients' attempts to reclaim power in medical encounters, stories constitute a significant factor in the healing process and therefore need to be taken seriously by doctors: "Patients must continually rewrite their life stories, incorporating illness. The process of doing this is a means of accepting a new reality. . . . So to interrupt a story is to interrupt a healing process" (1998:186). It is therefore necessary that doctors learn about the importance and functioning of narratives in everyday life and that they are sensitized to the power of dominant discourses about domestic violence by being exposed to the kinds of narratives transcribed and analyzed in this study.

On the other hand, doctors also need to learn how women think and feel about the problem. Domestic violence is still mostly neglected in medical training and rarely features in medical textbooks (García-Moreno 2002:1511). Campbell, who herself trains student nurses, emphasizes the importance of closing conceptual gaps at an early stage in the career of health care professionals, and she maintains that

> these realities are difficult for us and for students to understand. It is easier to categorize abused women in terms of pathological psychology and thereby distance oneself from a reality that may be only too close to home for female nursing students—which means most nursing students. Student attitudes can only be changed with dialog about these issues, sharing personal stories, and teaching about the wider context of the domination of women. The fact that woman battering is physical hitting and/or forced sex within a context of coercive control that crosses all domains of a woman's existence is a reality not captured by simply teaching this definition. Students need to get to know battered women personally in clinical experience and see role models of nurses conducting community advocacy for change. (1992:469)

Campbell implies that some nurses may have firsthand experience of a violent home or relationship and therefore feel reluctant to confront the problem in female patients. Other students may be too far removed from the lives some people suffer in order to fully understand and empathize with them. The main way to overcome such distances is by giving students the opportunity to meet victims and to exchange stories about their experiences. Since it might initially be difficult for students to become close to actual survivors of abuse, as Campbell argues, she first uses novels such as Walker's *The Color Purple* (1982), Morrison's *Beloved* (1987) and *Sula* (1982), Atwood's *The Handmaid's Tale* (1986), and Conroy's *The Prince of Tides* (1986) to expose students to the "realities" of domestic violence. Students are still able to "distance themselves—by putting the book down when necessary" (Campbell 1992:469), but they nonetheless form an initial impression of what experiencing violence can mean to a woman.

As I pointed out in chapter 2, medicine and narrative are not as far apart as we may at first imagine. To follow Hunter's (1991) line of reasoning, doctors' work can be regarded as "reading the patient as text," and it consists largely of interpreting the signs a patient presents with and of reformulating the interpretation in a specialized jargon, which makes a medical examination somewhat similar to literary studies. At the same time, GPs sometimes employ a narrative mode when talking to their patients in order to convey fairly complex medical terminology to a layperson. Doctors' diagnosis is also a retelling of the patient's own story of his or her illness in medical terms and entails the attachment of certain labels. The medical record, finally, presents the patient's case history and thus also follows a narrative pattern in the broadest sense. Although the "reliance on scientific observation, classification, and measurement and the sense of mastery associated with these activities, continues to define the parameters of much of medical practice," as Squier (1998:137) notes, a number of authors such as Hunter, Charon, and Coulehan (1995), Squier (1998), Rachman (1998), Charon (2005), and others have emphasized the importance of humanist and, more specifically, literary studies in the medical curriculum. The advantage of literary texts as a teaching device is that they offer an insight into the complexity of patients' lives, as Squier contends: "Indeed, the chief value of literature is the inherent complexity and holism of the story medium which reflects the complexity of real people living real lives, thereby allowing the student to reach a deeper and more comprehensive appreciation of the patient's predicament" (1998:131). There can be no doubt that the study of literary texts in the medical curriculum ultimately will not replace real encounters with patients and, in this case, with survivors of domestic abuse. Nevertheless, a narrative teaching module could contribute to students' acquisition of transferable skills such as communication and listening, knowledge of human nature and of the diversity of people's life experiences, lateral thinking, and the adoption and acceptance of other people's perspectives. Downie contends that "we learn from literature by imaginative identification with the situations or characters in literature, and by having our imaginations stretched through being made to enter into unfamiliar situations or to see points of view other than our own" (1991:96).

While the medical humanities and narrative medicine are only gradually making their way into British medical schools and are still largely absent from medical faculties in other Western countries, approximately 30 percent of American universities already offer literary teaching modules alongside courses in medical ethics and communication skills to medical students as part of a Humanities in Medicine course (Squier 1998:132). As Rachman points out, literature "has been used in medical instruction to promote moral and ethical reasoning, improve communication between doctor and patient, instill a deeper sense of medical history, explore the therapeutic value of storytelling, advance multicultural perspectives, and increase self-consciousness on the part of medical practitioners" (1998:123). More specifically, the study of literature and humanities in medicine fulfils three major functions, which are captured in the following conceptual approaches: the "ethical approach," the "aesthetic approach," and the "empathic approach" (Hunter, Charon, and Coulehan 1995:789). The ethical approach focuses on moral reflection and includes "images of healers in literature, cultural perspectives on illness, questions of justice in society, and the moral dimension of every patient-physician encounter." The aesthetic approach, by contrast, emphasizes "the literary skills of reading, writing, and interpretation, using them in the service of medical practice." In other words, students learn about their role as listeners to or readers of patients' stories and about strategies for interpreting and understanding these narratives. The aim is to encourage "tolerance for the ambiguity and turmoil of clinical situations." The empathic approach, finally, "aims to enhance the student's ability to understand the experiences, feelings, and values of other persons" (Hunter, Charon, and Coulehan 1995:789). Since language and narrative are indeed so central to medical practice, the sociolinguistic study of narrative is well placed to make the underlying linguistic mechanisms transparent to medical practitioners, and, similarly, the study of literature "makes the language of medicine, doctors, patients, and disease entities—the cultural frame of illness—visible" (Rachman 1998:123). This kind of narrative approach is useful if not imperative in the context of psychosocial problems such as domestic violence that require more than the kinds of treatment and help the biomedical model hitherto has to offer. It would also encourage cross-disciplinary collaboration, which, I would argue, is vital at a time when the rapidly accumulating amount of specialized knowledge in each single discipline poses the danger that experts in their respective field increasingly wear blinkers and thus perhaps miss important insights gained in other research areas.

What could a narrative teaching module in medicine look like? First, I think, it would be important to raise awareness among students about the importance of narrative in people's lives in general. Educators could, for example, alert students to this issue by drawing their attention to their own uses of narrative in their daily interactions with friends, family, and fellow students. Transcriptions of narratives as presented in this study and sociolinguistic narrative analysis would constitute core elements in this respect. This could be reinforced by short creative writing exercises in which students are encouraged to write little pieces concerning domestic violence. Charon (2005) demonstrates in what ways writing down their experiences can help (future) doctors sharpen their perceptions of past events, reinforce their attention to narrative detail in patients' stories, and thus ultimately help them affiliate with patients and colleagues. Students could also rewrite literary pieces from a new perspective, which, as Squier suggests, should be at least the point of view "of someone of a different race, gender, or age from the student" (1998:132). In order to bring their own possible uses of myths and stereotypes to the students' attention, it would be essential to make tools for narrative analysis available to them so they could understand the discursive mechanisms they themselves may unconsciously apply.

Since their own narratives might reflect only their own frustrations back to students and doctors, this preliminary stage should be followed by joint readings and discussions of literary and nonliterary texts that bring in the women's perspective. In the context of domestic violence, for example, we could add to the novels by Walker, Morrison, Atwood, and Conroy mentioned above Doyle's *The Woman Who Walked into Doors* and Fay Weldon's short story "Alopecia" (1981). More important, students and doctors should be acquainted with segments of women's stories about their encounters with GPs, especially with regard to what the women did not manage to say but expected the physicians to ask anyway. Data from empirical studies such as Williamson (2000) and Lawless (2001) could be used for such purposes.

Teachers could also include electronic narratives, which are available from a number of online forums and databases (McLellan 1997). The advantage of electronic narratives for physicians is, McLellan argues, that they are "a window on the ways illness can permeate lives and relationships, and on the ways the experience affects thinking and decision making. The texts often reveal truths that sick people and their families cannot or will not otherwise tell" (1997:1620). It is important to bear in mind that the discussions surrounding these texts ought to be relevant to whatever the course objective is. Thus, it would not make sense to undertake a close literary or discourse analysis with medical students if the goal was to teach them something about medical practice, or, as Squier puts it, "if the goal of a course is to further student understanding of patient and physician perspectives as part of the doctor-patient relationship course, asking students to discuss the uses of metaphors in a story or rhythm and alliteration in a poem may not advance, and may even divert attention from, this broad goal. On the other hand, if the goal is to develop a deeper understanding of how humans communicate, this kind of literary discussion may well be appropriate" (1998:133). Put another way, ethical and empathic approaches are sometimes to be favored over the aesthetic approach. Narrative and discourse analysis as they are applied in this study, however, ought to hold a central place in the training of student doctors, as they show up potential similarities and, more important, discrepancies between doctors' and patients' narratives. Furthermore, they offer useful tools for analyzing texts, since they unravel deeper cognitive processes and mechanisms of conceptualizing explanatory frameworks that contribute to the (re-)creation as well as the reinforcement of powerful and, very often, detrimental discourses about a topic such as domestic violence.

Ideally, already practicing GPs should be involved in some form of narrative teaching, although it would be more difficult for them to find the time and perhaps the motivation to attend seminars and workshops. The suggestions I make here at the very end of my study can only be a first offer to those interested in changing current medical training. There is simply not enough space in one book to also try and devise entire teaching modules.[2] This remains a task to be implemented in future research and policy making. I do hope, however, that this study will at least raise doctors' awareness by bringing to their attention the way they linguistically (re)construct their experiences with patients suffering domestic violence in their narratives and thus also the way they indirectly create knowledge and realities of the problem that can prove problematic in their daily practice work.

Appendix

The GPs' Narratives

This appendix includes complete transcriptions of all narratives, portions of which have been quoted earlier in the text.

Narrative 1

GP1: middle-aged male GP in a deprived area on the periphery of the city center

> J: Right. And do you think it affects any particular group in society?
>
> Dr.: No. It affects all groups of society. And I've had all groups of society in here. From social class one to social class six or five or whatever. A to Z or whatever the new sociological classifications are.
>
> J: Yeah, yeah. But, er, what, for example, about the difference between women and men. Do more women come in, men . . . ?
>
> Dr.: Uh, more women. As I say, **only this year I had my first two {males.}**
>
> J: {Men.} Aha. And do you find=
>
> Dr.: **=And [laughs] and, you know, one guy [has got a bigger] beating up than many women I have [come across].**

Narrative 2

GP2: young female GP in a city center practice

> J: Right. And looking back on all these years, what's your experience with domestic violence? Can you tell me about your experiences with domestic violence?
>
> Dr.: [?] You don't get an awful lot of people presenting with that as a problem, although a lot of women present [it] as a problem. It often comes out when you're speaking to them about something

else. Er, usually they'll come in 'cause [there's a] history, they're depressed, and sometimes it'll come out in that sort of situation. Or sometimes you'll— [sighs] **I'm thinking of one particular patient who brought her partner along with her. And it was quite clear, he was abusing her the whole way through, through my consultation. Verbally. You know, he was behaving in what I, I thought was a completely unacceptable [manner] all the way through in the interview. But I think he's probably, you know, he's probably an extreme case.** Er, so, it's probably very sporadic so you maybe don't, I wouldn't see a lot of people present with it. And, and if you do find it it tends to be rather an incidental thing you find rather than, than, er, something that stays [sort of] about there.

Narrative 2 (continued) and Narrative 3

GP2

J: Yes. You were talking about this couple, er, where the partner actually abused the woman in your practice. How did you react? I mean that must have been really=

Dr.: =Well, I just told, I said to him: "Excuse me, could you just shut up!" Because I was speaking to ... [It was just, er,] I wasn't alone. The health visitor commented on that and just, he was really very insulting to her but, she was having a baby with him. A previous relationship hadn't worked out. She very much wanted to make this one work. Um, she came from a fairly disrupted family background. Um, she's a vulnerable individual and [?] to go into this vulnerable situation. But you know, he was expecting her, while she was, she was heavily pregnant, to go and, he didn't wanna stay at her house, he wanted her to come up to his house and just being totally unacceptable. I told her that. I told her that he was treating her in an unacceptable way but she was just so laid back, "well ... " [mocking tone]. I don't think she saw it as, as a violent situation. But I thought what's [it] gonna take for people to, just to lash out at her. If it was just a situation like that and ...

J: Maybe many women just don't realize even, or they, they shut it out in a way because they don't want to see it.

Dr.: Yeah. Well, yes, if she's seen that was happening and if she's felt that she was being abused then she would have put this, she would have thought: "Gosh! I'm really stupid." And it would be easier for her to ignore it was happening or pretend it wasn't happening. And then she wouldn't feel so, so, you know, she maybe didn't feel so stupid. Although he's trying very hard to do it to her. And I, I, I can't quite figure out, I'm sure there's lots of individual factors that makes people stay with people that abuse them. And it's very difficult to tease them out. Um, if I, I mean I would never ever ever advise anybody to stay in that relationship. I just think that's just daft. **I remember the first time I saw it, quite cl——. I can still vividly remember the first time I came across a girl who'd been beaten by a guy and I was working in casualty. She was just a young girl and he'd, I just newly qualified, and this guy had hit her. And I said, [?] he had the house keys. Now then I said: "Could I have the house keys, please?" She wanted her flat keys. [And I said she wanted to be?] she just wanted to be here at the moment. And he got really, really, quite aggressive with me. And, fortunately there was police around and they got the keys and everything off him and, er, sat him down and told him to behave himself. I had a long chat with her, and she left with him. You know, she went back to him. I said: "Look, he's done that and you've forgiven him for once, he'll do it again to ya." And you just, I just wonder what happened, you know. But, you know, I thought, you know, if you let him do it this once [doctor knocks on the table with something] he'll always think he can get away with it again. And, she obviously, I don't know, I don't know why she went back.**

Narrative 4

GP3: late-middle-aged male GP in a city center practice

J: Yeah, yeah, coming back to the consultation, have you ever felt reluctant to ask a patient about, you know, whether there might be a problem with domestic violence?

Dr.: Reluctant only in terms of time constraints during a particular consultation. I mean if, if it's been going on for ages, er, and I know that it would be a can of worms that would be opened, I will maybe leave it . . . Only to make sure that there was an opening there to come back and discuss it further.

J: Right. Would it be the sensitivity of this issue=

Dr.: =I, I don't feel uncomfortable discussing these things with my patients. **I also had one man who was abused, by the way.**

J: Alright. Mmm. But that's surely not a very common case.

Dr.: **It's very unusual. But, I mean, cranky, I mean if I was [with a wife like this] [laughs], it's absolutely terrible.** Er, that's [?] No, I mean clearly it's, it's, it's . . . But I don't know, I, I have no personal difficulties about both bringing up the subject, er, about dealing with its potential, er, aftermath of that discovery.

Narrative 5

GP3

J: Mmm. Is there any case that is very vivid in your memory or, you know, which you can remember well?

Dr.: Um, I guess there are two or three but that's more because of, er, **I had one particular who's, who is, you know, in her second or third abusive relationship, er, and I, I just feel powerless, you know. I mean this woman by choice has sought out yet another person. Maybe not "sought out," I mean maybe it's that, er, her, her social, er, mix is with people who share that same, er, manner [?] to their previous partners. You know, if they're all boozers and they all meet in the pub or whatever then it's likely that she's gonna meet other people who, who are similar.** You know, in that we all tend to, um, find friendship with people who are or who have similarities. So it's, it's maybe not so surprising. But it's most surprising to me why people choose, er, to, to, to reenter, er, an arena of further physical violence having got out of a previous one. I find that really tough.

Narrative 6

GP4: female GP nearing retirement in practice near the university

J: Okay. And looking back on all these years, can you tell me a bit about your experiences with domestic violence?

Dr.: Um, well, not a lot. I'm not— not a lot is disclosed to you. Um, sometimes women come in with, er, injuries that they've sustained or sometimes they'll, er, you know, they'll come, er, for information about refuges and, er, things like that. But on the whole, er, not, not a lot presents to the GP. Um, sometimes you'll pick it, er, **I had a, I had, um, one girl who was particularly bad and her boyfriend broke her arm and she kept going back to him and, um, so, I knew quite a lot about her, um . . .**

Narrative 7 and Narrative 6 (continued)

GP4

J: Right. How about ethnic minorities? I could imagine you . . .

Dr.: I've got a lot of ethnic minorities. Again, um, I should have thought about this be———, um, **I've only had one family where I think there was violence. And, again it was very much, I think it did come out when the lady was very depressed and started to tell me about her, her problems, um, and, er, she actually, er, tried to commit suicide and that's when it came out then. Her husband was continually beating her up, um, maltreating her verbally and physically, so, and mentally,** [laughs] **I was upset as well. Er, but I, I think that was the only one . . .** But most of the ethnic people that I have here are university— um. I mean it is present in all, um, sectors of society but, um, again maybe more hidden if, er, with university . . . you know.

J: Yeah. Do you ever feel concerned you might not detect it {in a consultation?}

Dr.: {Yes, I think so.} Yeah. I think quite often I might suspect it. It's the same pro———possibly with child, um, um, vio———, er, er, violence to children. [Right]. **I was telling you about the girl with the broken arm. They have a small child and I suspect that the** child was maybe— er, and that was difficult because, you know, of course you have to bring the social workers in and things like that and that, I think that, er, concerns me more if that the children are involved as well in a violence. Um, but yes yes, I think they're probably, I, there is probably a lot that I don't pick up. Yes. Mmm. Mmm.

Narrative 8

GP4

J: Yeah. I mean that's something I can't imagine, you know, how you would react in that situation, um, because obviously it's a sensitive issue as well and I could imagine that you might not want to touch it, you know.

Dr.: Er, you were talking about ethnic, now, it's quite, um, it's quite difficult in ethnic becau——, er, because quite often the husband comes with the wife in an ethnic— In fact, I tell a lie, **I've seen it with one, well, that was a really bad one but there's a, a patient I've got at the moment and I think her husband mistreats her. And, um, um, the husband tends to come with the wife and of course she's not going to say that she's ...** so, it may be even more hidden in an ethnic grouping than it is in the Eu——, er, Western grouping. Yeah.

Narrative 6 (continued)

GP4

J: Have you ever seen people go back after {they've been here?}

Dr.: {Oh yes.} Yes, yes. **The girl that got her arm broke——, went, brok——, broken went back a few times but in the end she did leave but, er, I think it's because, er, danger of the child in the end of the day that made the difference [for her], um.** I've also had people who have been in one violent relationship and then have gone into another violent relationship and then that, that really is a thing that they need to unlearn [laughs], you know, what kind of partners you choose, which again is often quite difficult. Maybe assertiveness training and, er, things like that ...

Narrative 9

GP4

J: Okay. Um, what do you think about the status of domestic violence in the whole health setting or the National Health Service, for example? Do you think it's maybe neglected?

Dr.: I think it probably is given a, given a low status, um. I'm just thinking, I was in G-Docs, er, just a few weeks ago, and, er, I was called out to something with, you know, that was a domestic violence situation. Um, it was kind of given a lower status than or a low——, lower priority than say, maybe an elderly person with a stroke or a heart attack or something like that. So, you know, it was kind of a nuisance that we had to go out and see it and, er, then they got the social workers involved and I say I think they kind of think, "Well, it's the social workers' problem, it's not ours," you know, and the police were involved as well, so, they left it with the social workers, so. Poor social workers, that's not fair [laughs].

Narrative 10 and Narrative 11

GP5: early middle-aged female doctor in a student health practice

J: Right. Looking back on your experience before student health, is there any case that you vividly remember or . . . ?

Dr.: Um . . . the ones I remember at the moment are more, it's more, you wanted domestic violence as opposed to child, the violence towards children? Um, I can't remember, I should have thought about this before you came, um . . . No, I can't, sorry. I'll be thinking about it as we're talking.

J: Yeah. Okay. Um, well, if someone comes in with signs of domestic violence=

Dr.: =Oh, I do remember. I do remember. An amazing case. Yes, I had an amazing case in casualty once when, um, somebody had, um, that was a long time ago, somebody had come in and obviously had been, you know, really quite badly beaten up and was terrified to, to go home. And her partner arrived in casualty at the front door, demanding to see her. Um, and we didn't know what to do really and what we did, we phoned Women's Aid and we spoke to this amazing lady who has now retired. She was a, a professor's wife at the hospital, um, and she arranged everything. And she, it was almost as the cloak-and-dagger stuff, she appeared in the back door and smuggled this woman out. Then she went to the hostel.

J: What did you feel at that time, I mean . . . ?

Dr.: Well, it was quite, och, I think, the problem was that we never knew what happened. You know, you never know how, how things turned out in the long term. Um, we had another case here actually. That's, that, we had a little girl who was a drug addict and her boyfriend was a drug addict and that was really sad and she was coming in with black eyes and, you know, bruises and all sorts of things and she was different in that she just couldn't do anything about it. You know, no matter what we suggested she . . . wasn't able to, to break away from this guy. Unless while he was in prison, which was alright, she was much better then and she just, she didn't finish her degree and she just looked iller and iller and more and more tired and eventually she just disappeared and we don't know what's happened to her. She left Aberdeen and goodness knows where she is now.

Narrative 12

GP6: *late-middle-aged male doctor in an affluent area near the city center*

J: Okay. Um, can you think of any particular story a patient came up with or . . . ? Is there any case that's very vivid in your memory, for example?

Dr.: Um, yes, there was a wife of a taxi driver who was, er, accused of, er, rape. Er, he used to, er, take female passengers, [first of all there was alcohol and drugs] and ended up being caught and eventually in prison. Um, during the court proceeding she was generally reasonably supportive, I mean, saying that they shouldn't have raised these allegations that [?] that, er, settled down when she was, er, away, um, they split up and, er, when he came out of prison again she wouldn't let him back into her house, er, initially. Eventually he came back into the house and, er, she ended up leaving and moving into a hostel with her kids. Um, and she was a, you know, nice, decent person. Obviously [being very hot-burnt with these . . .] That's a, an unusual case maybe. Um, there's always a lot of unhappiness in relationships and when, um, people are obliged for all sorts of reasons to stay together I think the situation is worse. Er, if the woman is dependent on the male provider then it's a lot more difficult for them to move out of the situation. More women will leave men than men will leave women.

Narrative 13

GP6

Dr.: And learned behavior from their own childhoods that hurts, a lot of child abuse and, er, sexual abuse. Er, you look back and see it happened there over generations. **Um, I had a patient who, um, er, had been sexually abusing his children, both boys and girls and, when he died, I was quite surprised when his, when the kids expressed pleasure that he'd actually died. But the father himself had been abused in childhood. This is the sort of violent behavior [that goes back for] generations.** Er, if there is a history in the family it'll repeat itself down in generations [?]. Learned, learned behavior.

Narrative 14

GP7: male doctor nearing retirement working with the homeless

J: Yeah. Um, is there any case that's particularly vivid in your memory, anything that was . . . ?

Dr.: **I think possibly, er, the one and only time I've ever come across a, um, an abused man. Because I'd read about them but it took me completely [by] surprise when I actually met one because he was a big-bellied chap who actually ran away from Dundee and allegedly a very small, er, wife who did, er, exhibit, er, violence towards him.** And again I couldn't understand, er, [I'll] never be able to understand why [you have to use] violence in a relationship but I couldn't understand why he accepted it for so long but again, there was, he was a chap on the road. I didn't see him for very long, I never established the truth of the situation. Or maybe . . . Yes, it's, er, it's often been surprising to me, er, people I've known for a long, long time, who've seemed like very decent, er, people, very, er, decent families, decent relationships, and all of a sudden out of the blue they emerge maybe after fifteen, twenty years, perhaps even from a, a son or daughter that, er, the violent relationship or "Dad had been beating up mum for a long time!" and, er, she put up with it and kept quiet. So, it, it can be extremely surprising, it's, you, you're often lightyears away from guessing that it might be a problem.

Narrative 15

GP8: late-middle-aged male doctor in a student health practice

J: Is there any case that's particularly vivid in your memory?

Dr.: There was one girl, yeah, that was pinned to a wall and had her head bashed in, and by someone, er, another student, um, and she was terrified and it definitely affected her in a bad way, I mean, she, um, she left [?] and the person that assaulted her, that was an atrocious sight. She was bigger than me, I remember that. That's the most, that's the only one that has been in the last seven years where there was a real problem, you know, where there was a, a difficult outcome, if you like. The rest, they were all minor. And then in general practice, general work in here, um, well, there's quite a few, really, I mean, it's, 'cause none of these stood out because they were just, um, commonly, um, you know, nothing, well, none of these stood out in the sense that they didn't, you know, bother me a lot. They maybe came with a bruise [and that] and you don't, you didn't really know what the outcome was unless they were divorced or something.

Narrative 16

GP8

J: Do you ever feel concerned that you don't detect it? [?] or . . .

Dr.: No, I think if people complain about something, I think, I'm reasonably aware that I [could pick it up] that there's a problem or that there might be a problem and you can obviously ask. Not, people may not come. I think there's a hidden, huge hidden, you know, mass of it that no one comes forward and I've never known of a male being assaulted but I know that men do get assaulted by their wives. **I have a friend who was assaulted by his wife. So, I know it happens. And, er, he was, er, he was kicked and various other things, um, and he ended up arrested. Incredibly, even though I'm sure I know that it was her who assaulted him. She admitted it, you know, and he was arrested.** I just find this, feminism's just gone completely bananas as far as I am concerned.

Narrative 17

GP8

J: Do you think that some GPs maybe ignore the issue?

Dr.: Yep, because they're people, because they're men, because they're under stress, because there might be a woman who's been brought up in a very sheltered environment and hasn't got a clue how low people live their life, yes, I think [?]. And there's all sorts of reasons for that. I think it's, yeah, I don't know. It's tricky. But I think people, GPs will ig——, I think, doctors [?]. Some doctors are far better than others at communicating with patients. Communication is not something that you were taught at medical school much when I went to medical school. It might be taught more now. You weren't even taught to look somebody in the [eyeball], you know. [To look in the eyeball of] somebody [can] help you really understand what's going on, you know. If you sit and look at the desk when they're speaking to you— **and I had a partner who did that, and I'm sure he couldn't really be empathic with any of his patients— not because he was a bad person because he wasn't, but he just couldn't look at them.** You have to give, you have to make people think you're interested or they won't come back. Would you agree?

J: Yeah, I think so. I think communication skills are very important . . .

Dr.: Yeah.

J: Mmm.

Narrative 18

GP8

And, I [always] think that it's going a wee bit too far, you know, when, I [can give you a really good little story.] Well, on Radio 4, about five, six months ago, there was this news broadcast when this, two kids were seen standing outside a school talking to a man, right? Now, people saw this man talking to, [the] man seemed to be talking to these children [who were] about nine, right, or whatever, and they phoned the police. And the police came [?] with the blue light flashing to the school, and the kids had gone. And the man had gone, so they went, they went into the school and they couldn't find out who these two kids were but, so they ended up doing a, a roll call, I think, and all the kids were there, fine, no problem, and somebody said to the police they'll actually, [what] will they charge him with anyway, is, can a man not speak to children? Now, it's, it makes a point, that story. A very big point. You can't make outright assumptions that men are bad, right? Even in domestic violence situations, it, it's not right. It's [?] you get the hysterical one, um, you know, to assume things in society. This is not how the world is. The world is much subtler than that and I, I know I wouldn't deny for a minute that most emotional possibly, certainly the most visible violence, domestic violence, is perpetrated by men on women. I wouldn't deny that. I think it's grossly oversimplistic, I think, that that's the only issue there.

Narrative 19

GP9: middle-aged male GP in a suburban practice

J: Right. Is there any case that's particularly vivid in your memory?

Dr.: No. [laughs]

J: No.

Dr.: I'm not very helpful there. Um, no, as I say, it's not an issue that I've been dealing with very much of lately anyway so there's nothing very fresh, er, um, there's, I mean in twenty-five years you're going to see an amount of this but it isn't, it isn't a major part of my work. **We've had, I'm only aware of one fatality from domestic violence and that was through alcohol and, the chap's now locked up.**

J: Alright. Did that end really badly?

Dr.: **That was not good. [?] And there were, he didn't realize that she was dead until he sobered up and she had the head in the fireplace. That was unpleasant.**

J: Oh, God, how do you react as a GP when something like this happens, I mean . . . ?

Dr.: **Well, um, supportively but I thought that, I mean, you know, he declaring that it must have been an accident but, in fact, eventually he was arrested and taken away.**

Narrative 20

GP9

I think it is mainly, er, mainly to do with, with, with sexual domestic partners as being the, the center of it. Clearly, it extends beyond that to, to families and so on. Um, I, that's my, my sort of, um, "view" of it, and I don't think in terms of sibling-sibling, I know that's been a common thing, um, clearly parent-child would be another sort of violence which is difficult to, or indeed child-parent for the elderly but, um, again, these are things that we don't see very much of or at least don't recognize. Granny bashing and child battering are not something that we see a lot of, and again, maybe we miss some of it, I'm sure we do.

J: {Similar to . . .}

Dr.: {Similar to} male-female, yeah.

J: Right.

Dr.: **And the last person I had in who'd been complaining of being hit was actually a man who was complaining that his girlfriend had been beating him up. So . . . [laughs]**

Narrative 21

GP10: middle-aged female GP in a deprived city center area

J: Mmm. Mmm. So, what would you suggest to this person, you know, I mean, once domestic violence has been established in a consultation, what would your next step be or . . . ?

Dr.: Um, I mean I usually make sure that, that their physical, again, it depends very much on what's been presented to me, as I say, it, it, och, **the most recent things that I remember is actually people who had got to that stage where they wanted to involve the police and therefore needed a catalog of injuries in case they have to do anything with it, you know, and that's a sensible thing that has to be done.** And it's, it's a distracting thing as well. You can do that while chatting and [?], so the physical thing has to be dealt with.

Narrative 22

GP11: young male GP in a deprived area on the outskirts of the city

J: Mmm, mmm, right. Is there any case that's particularly vivid in your memory?

Dr.: **I've had one lady who's, er, she works in a [?] major department store in town and she's come in with sort of facial bruising and then having to go to work. Or, at some point in the week going to work. So, you know, it's, er, sad, sad for her because then everyone else realizes what's, er, or, [?].**

J: Yeah.

Dr.: But, I mean I've never seen a real major, er, domestic abuse apart from in, where I was working in casualty years ago.

Narrative 23

GP12: late-middle-aged male GP in an area on the outskirts of the city center

J: Yeah, yeah, I mean, what are the reasons for domestic violence anyway, why does it happen?

Dr.: Um, well, I, I think drink often is, is a case and if, um, and if you compound that with the man having, um, not, not being a negotiator of problems but just, just doing that so then, I suppose, at the end of the day, because, because we all, we all have our own rit——, rituals in, in our relationships, then, you know, if, if the woman nags or gets on to someone and he, you know, he hits it back and, it's actually trying to change people's behavior patterns is very difficult so, so there may be a, you know, a, just a sort of fixed pattern in behavior and in a relationship that goes like that so, um, I suppose sex— you know, sexual, er, demands or refusals come into it as well, um, some people just, husbands may like, some of them, they seem to like the power of, you know, of doing that. Um, and [?] I suppose, it's, er, they're even sort of, a degree of sadomasochism, that some people actually like being beaten up, er, [?]. **I mean I had a, a, I mean a patient many years ago and she, I mean she used to come in and reg——, regale us with the, the most bizarre and, er, tales of terrible sadomastics, masochistic stuff and, but she stayed with her husband for ten years, you know, um, er, it was, um, you know, it, it was, it was almost sort of schizoid that, you know, she was, she'd sit there and say, "He's doing this, that and the other," you know, "[took] me and beat up" and "Why don't you leave?" "Oh, I can't leave!"** [laughs], you know . . .

Narrative 24

GP13: middle-aged female GP in a deprived area on the outskirts of the city

J: Mmm. Do you find that your patients often go back to the same situation?

Dr.: Yeah.

J: Yeah?

Dr.: They don't come out of it, yeah. Or they, they are pregnant and go back or, **I can think of one woman who, you know, clearly that was why she was so upset and [everything] and got her through that but she wouldn't leave him. That was an older woman, you know, now middle-aged [?]. The stigma attached to all the family and relations, she couldn't extract herself out of that.** And it's quite a thing for a woman of that age to become single again and live on her own despite the abuser's [?] it's very difficult . . .

Narrative 25

GP13

J: Yeah [skeptical facial expression]. [both laugh] It's been going on for so long and now you wonder if anything could be done.

Dr.: I know.

J: It's quite depressing.

Dr.: It is. It is. I know, um, I don't know why it should be. It's to do with power, I'm sure, in men [?] power and frustration and ways of communicating that. [pause] Yeah. But sometimes the women do get out and a very, very old lady [?] terrible test and she eventually learned to allow her husband in our sympathies. [?] how, I mean, she'll be fine 'cause, I mean, she must have been terribly lonely 'cause this house was away from, er, all social network but she put up with him for years and, er, she's quite well. And [?] she walked out on her own but she did it, you know. It took her years and years. I mean, she took herself another house [?].

Narrative 26

GP14: young female GP in a deprived area on the outskirts of the city

J: Mmm. Do you find that women often go back as well?

Dr.: Yeah, yeah. I mean I've got one in particular who, her husband, um, is an alcoholic and is abusive and aggressive towards her and now towards her baby, er, use, you know, sort of uses her as a, as a weapon. And she has tried to leave him and has got an injunction against him but then has changed her mind and just gone back to him again. And there's not much more I can do in that scenario really, which I find very difficult 'cause she's still upset about it and she's still affected by it so . . .

Narrative 27

GP14

J: Mmm. And once you've got a suspicion, how would you proceed, I mean, how would you pursue the issue?

Dr.: I would basically just sort of say directly, you know, "Is, is there problems at home? Are you having problems with your partner or your family?" and, you know, "What exactly is happening? Do they hit you? Do they shout at you?" Sometimes it's not even just, I mean, you can have families where, yes, the husband's perhaps abusive towards the wife, he can be verbally abusive, but you sometimes find even the kids are like that as well. **I had one woman whose grown-up kids have just seen the father be like this and they were not physically aggressive but, um, mentally aggressive towards their mother all the time, quite threatening and, um, again, that's a horrible situation if your whole family seems to be getting on at you and giving you a hard time. It's, it's not very good.** I, I'm usually sort of fairly direct asking them, sometimes they actually quite want to speak about it. They can't speak to anyone else.

Narrative 28

GP14

J: Um, a number of GPs I've interviewed have said that time might be a problem, that they might not want to broach the subject because obviously you're only on ten minutes or something and then it might be difficult to open this "can of worms."

Dr.: Um, I would tend to ask them anyway, um, and if there's a hint of something and we start getting involved, **um, I had one girl who, ach, she had a horrible family. She, her, her mother told her when she was [?], she was about eighteen, that her father wasn't her father and "either way, that's your father over there." And so she'd become very confused and I tried to approach him** and then, a year or so later, the mother said: "That was all a lie, he's not your father at all, blah blah blah" and there was a whole big [discussion] in the families and she was very upset about it. You know, she was dressed, she set to work, when you actually went into it, and you really had to go into that in detail, but I said to her: "Well, you know, we've cer——, I've just [been] speaking for about twenty minutes. [I'm kind of] running out of time." So, get her to come back and some will come back, some won't. She did come back but, um, you do have to give them the chance to say it. And if you don't pick up the cues then they just maybe never come to the surface again, you know. So I would, I would tend to ask and then, if need be, get them to come back. Um, I tend to do that.

Narrative 29

GP15: middle-aged male GP in a suburban area

J: Yeah. How do you feel anyway when you encounter domestic violence? Do you ever feel upset, for example?

Dr.: I think you always do. I think there's rarely a situation when you don't. But sometimes [tempered] if, um, **we've got, um, one couple in the practice who are both, um, alcoholics and she's the victim of, um, violence, um, and you, ach, I don't know, and it always seems to happen when they're on a [bender] but, um, but, er, he hits her, he punches her and kicks her and [pause] and you still, I, I think you still feel sympathy for, for what's happened but, um, I think it's frustration as much as anything, you think, "Well, why do they do that? Why stay on? Why keep drinking?" but, you know, it's, it's, it's, it's their life really. That's the way it's always been, and it isn't something that can be changed usually [?].** But I think you always do feel sorry for the victim of any violence, whether it's male or female or whatever the circumstances, human nature, I suppose.

Narrative 30

GP16: middle-aged male GP in practice in the wider city area near the university

J: Okay. Well, first of all, thank you very much for giving me your time because, as you can imagine, it's not easy for me to get doctors to talk to me=

Dr.: ={Probably.}

J: {Many of} them say they don't have time, others say it's not an issue for them. So I wanted to ask you: Do you think domestic violence is an issue for GPs?

Dr.: Er, well, I think it, unfortunately, I think, it probably is because, I mean, **this morning alone, I've had a patient in who has trou-**

ble with the family. It's a difficult one to, to best try to manage [?]. Yes, so I've had a patient fairly recently and I've had one or two of them in the past and, er, I find it difficult to know how best to manage them 'cause where to send them and how to get their best, where do they get their best advice, and, er, 'cause it's not something I can do a lot about except encouraging to seek advice from appropriate sources.

Narrative 30 (continued)

GP16

Dr.: Yeah. I'm sure there's a lot hidden, yeah. I mean, a lot of women won't admit to it, but if they came in with black eyes, you know, obvious bruising, then, er, I think, I will confront them a bit about it and discuss it and see what happened to this lady, for example.

J: Mmm. Can you tell me a bit about . . . ?

Dr.: About this lady?

J: Yeah.

Dr.: She, well, she's interesting. She's a schiz——, she's labeled as a schizophrenic but she's not, she's not really, she's not, er, particularly bad in that way and she lives, um, in a flat she has bought and she has a partner who she wants to get out of the flat, who's really ins——, er, installed himself in there and [has lived] there for a number of years and, um, he, er, er, he's, er, mentally and physically abusive towards her and, um, he really just, er, pushes her around and makes her do all the shopping, he makes her carry everything, he turns off all the lights and the telly when he wants it off, he changes the TV program if he doesn't like it on and he resorts to physical violence and, and she came in the other week, last week, with a big black eye and some bruising and then I had a chat with her about it and, er, [she felt ashamed] and then, before I suspected it I'd never actually known that he's been physically abusive but, er, she obviously is unhappy with him but can't get him out of the flat. He pays rent and he's fairly, er, aggressive [?]. She likes to watch some television program, he prefers if she puts it, the, the nasty, aggressive things on the telly. So she's in a bit of a dilemma and, being mentally unwell, she, she hasn't worked for a number of years, she doesn't have, um, she, she's not very skilled at times to organi——, to manage this situation. She does have support from the CPN [clinical psychiatric nurse] but I don't think, er, it's very difficult to know how best to help her actually 'cause I said to her last week she should go to, to seek legal advice. I suggested that she maybe goes to the Citizens Advice first to get some help with that. She's not, well, financially, she's badly off so she's worried about all sorts of legal fees. I suggested to her that one option might be to come out of the flat and seek refuge and then [the Citizens Advice section] will get him out but she understandably is reluctant to do that because it's her flat, she actually pays the mortgage and he pays her rent. That's pretty minimal but he does. So she's in a very unhappy situation and she really doesn't want to get involved with him but she can't get rid of him.

J: Alright. But she was fairly up front about the {problem?}

Dr.: {Very, yeah.} Well, I've known her for quite a, about ten years so she and, er, with her schizophrenic illness it's taken a while getting her to talk about things but she's actually quite well from that point of view, she's not psychotic at all at the moment and I don't think, er, that's an issue. I think there's an issue in that she is not very good at managing the situation and, and she's, and she's not working, she's only forty-six but she's not working. She has no other financial, er, input of actual benefits. Um, but I mean it was obvious when she had the black eye that, that she'd been assaulted but she was quite moved from that how it happened and she did say this wasn't a new thing, it happened several times in the past.

Narrative 31 and Narrative 30 (continued)

GP16

But, er, so it really depends on how, how sure you are that, in your own mind, that things are wrong at home or with the partner.

But I've had a few come in with relatives, you know, son, grown-up sons bringing their mothers in to say that she wouldn't come along but "I'm bringing her along because her boyfriend's beating her up" or, or stepfather, "My stepfather is beating her up" or that kind of, and that, you know, that's another way of presenting. The family eventually having had enough of it and saying a word, you know, telling you about it over the phone and expecting you to then bring it up with the patient when they come in. So, there are different ways of getting to . . .

J: Mmm, mmm, yeah. Some of the GPs I've interviewed so far have mentioned time as a problem, that it might be difficult because you have ten minutes or {something.}

Dr.: {It's very difficult,} yeah. The only way is to get them to come back and, er, er, I mean, this lady with schizophrenia, I saw her last week, I've seen her this week and she's coming back in two weeks and I've suggested that she better try to, I might get and see [her] back in again and see what's wrong. I don't hold that much hope for her 'cause I don't think she's actually going to get her act together and try and do anything but I have documented the intrusion and I have said to her I'd be willing to support her, you know, if she gets in touch with a lawyer that I can come forward with what she's told me today and, er, the injuries she's presented with. But time is difficult, I know that well. And we're referring on to, I suppose, other agencies, I mean, er, er, that's, that's, that's the other thing is knowing who to refer on to. Again, you have to get the patient to comply with that and actually get in touch.

Narrative 32

GP17: young female GP in a wider city area practice

J: Right. Okay, but can you tell me a bit about the experiences you've had?

Dr.: Um, [sighs] my interview is probably flavored by the fact that I've actually been asked to speak on domestic violence in pregnancies, up at the maternity hospital 'cause I'm the antenatal doctor here and I was asked to come and do a presentation. So I kind of asked around and spoke to the midwives, spoke to the health visitors to pick out a few families that they thought there was something going on and so I did this sort of mini-audit of their notes. Um, so, I suppose, there was one girl in particular I remember her being really quite a hard thing for me. She was always at the surgery, minor, usually minor, minor complaints or she'd drag along her little boy and it'd be something very minor with him, um, and they were here all the time and then, one day, basically she admitted that, you know, I, I'd actually visited her at home as well, in the presence of this very "loving" in inverted commas boyfriend and then one day she admitted to me that he'd been abusing her for years but her son was out of, as a result of a rape, and it was just horrendous. Now, since that has come up I have never, I see her once a year. So, in the long run, I've saved a lot of time and she's perhaps, she's got rid of the boyfriend which was the real cure, there was nothing medical I could do for her, um, but that really sticks in my mind, that case.

Narrative 33

GP17

J: Right. Do you think domestic violence is an issue for any other group?

Dr.: Um, I don't know if it is, I suppose that we're a bit slanted up here in Aberdeen but I just get the impression that some ethnic minorities perhaps, maybe not so much in the way of physical violence but actually psychological dominance by the males within the family, I mean that's maybe a cultural norm for them. I can think of one situation where I've got a Bangladeshi family who's had, the husband is, is incredibly overpowering, um, to such an extent, this very intelligent woman who has her own job and, and, you know, runs the home, the job, and the children still doesn't really make any decisions on her, her own life. I don't

know if you could classify that as violence. I think she's very,
very dominated by what her husband says, er . . .

J: Yeah, it's more like verbal abuse mainly . . .

Dr.: Yeah. And I think certain, you know, in certain cultures perhaps
the women are less perhaps likely to come and, and see, open up to
the, to ma——, you know, to the, um, health visitor or GP or
whatever.

Narrative 32 (continued)

GP17

J: So it's really a question of awareness . . .

Dr.: Awareness, that's the big one.

J: Yeah.

Dr.: Mmm. But part of me also makes me think, and it's perhaps unfair, but part of me makes me think that I wish women had the
confidence and tell us if there was a problem. I sometimes feel,
you know, you're taking this for so long, you know, it's part, I
suppose part of it is building up a relationship with all your patients and, so they trust you and will come to you with problems
but, **I mean, especially the girl that I, I was talking about, if she
told me even a year earlier, you know, and I just wish she had
'cause I felt like I had a good rapport with her and I felt like she
trusted me, um, I certainly had a lot of contact with her and I
feel why couldn't, maybe it was my fault that she couldn't say**
but sometimes I feel women should, I mean I know their self-
esteem and their confidence has been shattered for many, many
years but I just wish they would feel that they could come and
tell us if there was a problem, 'cause we're not gonna bandy it
about, you know, if it's totally confidential. We can give them advice. If they don't want to take our advice, fine, but I wish they
would let us, er, let us know. And I just wish that, you know,
there's been a few adverts on the telly recently and it's quite good,
domestic violence [funds] and, um, but I wish there was more
in the magazines, in the media to make it acceptable for women
to go and ask for help. It's hard enough to do anyway but we're

not mind readers and if we're having a busy surgery and, all we see is the pink page in front of us. We're not looking through notes all the time and analyzing everybody's consultation. So, if they come in with a sore throat we deal with their sore throat and then they go but if they just gave us some, some better clues.

J: Yeah. But maybe they feel they=

Dr.: =but maybe they are giving us clues. Sorry. [laughs]

J: Maybe they just feel they can't bother you with this problem {because}

Dr.: {I know.}

J: because they might not see it as a medical {problem}.

Dr.: {problem}. Yeah, but it is, they should, they should be educated so they know that they can come and, and see us.

Narrative 34

GP17

J: Yeah. Do you think that's maybe a shortcoming?

Dr.: [takes a deep breath] Yes, definitely but I think especially working in A&E [accident and emergency] and the amount of women we saw, **I had, er, a girl who, oh, it was so strange, who was, she, the story was she'd fallen down the stairs and at the bottom of the stairs there was a glass door. She'd fallen down the stairs and through the door and her leg was in ribbons and I sat about an hour stitching it up, and her husband was a drug [user] and he sat with me, the whole hour, saying sweet things in her ear, you know, and, you know, being generally supportive and so nice and so kind. And then when she came back to the dressing clinic, to st——, to have her stitches out and see how her leg was doing, she admitted that he'd actually pushed her through a glass door and that he'd been violent towards her for a long time.** But he wasn't, you know, he obviously wasn't there, um, at that point. So, that was great she told me and that gave me great in——, insight into what's been happening but I felt then totally unprepared to do anything about it. I mean I did nothing. I

did nothing. I sympathized with her, I sent her on her way because, you know, we hadn't been told, I mean there's the A&E
training but nobody ever mentioned issues of domestic violence. Perhaps they do now, that was, um, ten years ago.

Narrative 35

GP19: young male GP in an affluent suburban area

J: Mmm. Do you think that the women in South Africa were more
up front about it? I mean, did they come out fairly quickly? You
say you saw it more than you see it here? Maybe it's also an issue
of coming out? I don't know.

Dr.: Well, I think their violence was more obvious, you know, if someone breaks his wife's arms then that obviously is an obvious issue. And I'm talking about these kind of things, you know. **Um,
I had a once a woman where the, her son had a, an acute psychotic attack because her husband was, had been pointing a gun
at her and things like this. So that, or, you know, rape and things
like this, really horrendous things and then it is just obvious.**
Um, otherwise, I don't think so, I don't, I don't, I don't think African, Africans are at all up front about many things that Europeans are up front about and the other way round. So they're up
front about different issues and, er, and in African society you
don't talk much about issues that are related to sexuality, for instance, and things that happen between husband and wife. So,
no, I don't think they're up front about it. It's just that sometimes
it's so obvious that, that you can't hide it.

Narrative 36

GP20: late-middle-aged female GP in an affluent area near the city center

J: Right, mmm. Can you tell me a bit about your experiences with
patients who suffered domestic violence?

Dr.: It doesn't seem to happen very often but, but, I mean, it, it does
happen a lot, I know that, um, patients don't always present with
it that often. **I mean I remember, this was years ago, my worst
patient came up with bruise marks all round her neck and she**

was quite open about it and she came in and said: "I'd just like you to make a note of all these injuries because my husband tried to strangle me yesterday and, um, I, I just want you to all note it because I'm going to sue hi——, I'm going to take him to court" or whatever. She was very up front about it. Um, but mostly it's, it's the, the scenario that things aren't, that the patients have said things aren't going well and they'll tell you that the, their partner sometimes hits them, say, when they're drunk or, or that sort of thing. Sometimes they'll tell you in retrospect, you know, that they've left him because obviously he was just "lifting the hand," that's always what they say up here. "He was lifting his hand and, um, that's why I left." And, um, that's quite common as well that they sometimes don't want to tell you actually at the time. Sometimes they do.

Notes

1. Introduction

1. General practitioners (GPS) are equivalent to family medicine practitioners in the United States.

2. Narrative

1. I must add the caveat that the Sapir-Whorf hypothesis has come to be known in two versions, the "weak" and the "strong": "According to the strong version, people's cognitive categories are determined by the languages they speak. According to the weak form, people's behavior will tend to be guided by the linguistic categories of their languages under certain circumstances" (Fasold 1990:53). Although the strong version in particular has received much criticism, the Sapir-Whorf hypothesis has been neither fully accepted nor entirely rejected. Nevertheless, since language at least to a certain degree conditions people's conceptualizations of social problems and, indeed, of the world around them, we can turn the argument on its head and maintain that the analysis of language is important in order to uncover the subtler mechanisms that facilitate such conditioning.

2. For a general discussion of misunderstandings and their consequences see Hinnenkamp (1998). Examples of how miscommunication can lead to fatal events like plane crashes are provided in Cushing (1990, 1994). Another area in which the impact of language has featured prominently is forensic linguistics. Tiersma and Solan (2002) provide a good overview of this study area. For examples of the significance of linguistic expertise in court trials see Labov and Harris (1994) and Shuy (1993).

3. Zimmerman and Boden argue along the same lines when they propose "structure-as-interaction" as a "way of articulating the agency/structure intersection": "Members can and must make their actions available and reasonable to each other and, in so doing, the everyday organization of experience *produces* and *reproduces* the patterned and patterning qualities we have come to call social structure. The organization of talk displays the essential reflexivity of action and structure and, in so doing, makes available what we are calling structure-in-action" (1991:18, 19, emphasis in original).

4. The terms *orientation* and *complicating action* are derived from Labov and Waletzky (1967) and are clarified in chapter 3.

5. Narratology originally began as a more generalist approach, the models of which

were claimed to be universally applicable, regardless of what shape the narrative took (Prince 1997:39). More recently, authors have put forward integrative approaches that take into consideration not only aspects of "classical" narratology and discourse linguistics but also perspectives on narrative borrowed from cognitive psychology and artificial intelligence (Herman 1997, 1999b, 2001; Jahn 1999; Nünning and Nünning 2002a, 2002b). These "new" approaches emphasize the contextual and processual nature of narrative and thereby overcome the dilemmas of purely structuralist analyses, which, no matter how accurate and detailed, always convey a sense of incompleteness.

6. Research on language use in the courtroom undertaken by Lind and O'Barr (1979) shows that the distribution of "power and powerless speech" indeed influences jurors' judgment and evaluation of witnesses giving testimony, on the one hand, and attorneys, on the other. "Powerless speech," that is, speech marked, among other things, by frequent use of intensifiers ("very," "so," "too," etc.), hypercorrect grammar, polite forms, hedges ("kinda," "I guess," "well," etc.), and rising intonation, was found to make witnesses appear less favorable socially, especially if they were male. Similarly, test subjects considered "fragmented" testimony more negative than "narrative" testimony: "When differences do occur in reactions to narrative and fragmented testimony they are in the direction of more favourable evaluations of witnesses giving narrative answers" (Lind and O'Barr 1979:79).

7. Bruner refuted this dichotomy in his 2003 book *Making Stories*, not so much in the sense that he disclaimed the existence of the narrative and the paradigmatic modes of thinking but in that he reformulated their relationship. While in his earlier writings Bruner regarded the narrative mode as translatable into the scientific mode (and thus as subsidiary to it), he now claims that narrative thinking in fact shapes our perceptions of the world and is thus the starting point of all knowledge.

8. In Linde's example a subordinate not only informs her boss about an incident of violence perpetrated by one client on another but also relates the actions taken by herself and her colleagues to restore institutional order. Thus, her narrative in a sense recreates policy as well as notions of institutional mission and power relationships.

9. It is interesting to note in this context that the development of the "institutional memory" of domestic abuse in the social sciences also changed over the years, moving from virtual nonexistence in the 1950s and early 1960s (Gelles 1980; Hague and Wilson 2000) to a proliferation of research in the 1990s (Johnson and Ferraro 2000). In recent years the issue has become more topical in social science studies, which can be seen in the extensive research presented in articles and monographs (Dell and Korotana 2000; Mooney 2000; Radford, Friedberg, and Harne 2000; Hague et al. 2002; Mezey et al. 2002), research projects undertaken in Britain, for example (Coid et al. 2001; Richardson et al. 2001, 2002; Bradley et al. 2002); and journals specifically dealing with this issue (*Violence against Women*; the *Journal of Interpersonal Violence*).

10. In her study on protective order interviews with Latina survivors of abuse Trinch shows how both victims and interviewers employ euphemisms to evade a direct discus-

sion of the topic of marital rape during the interviews and thus reconstruct inaccurate accounts of abusive relationships. This ultimately also falsifies the reports and statistical material that constitute the institutional memories of the district attorney's office and the pro bono law clinic investigated: "Thus, the statistical data they have compiled are at best incomplete, and at worst, completely misleading" (Trinch 2002b:600).

11. The findings can be summarized by quoting the Tayside Women and Violence Group: "Agencies do not offer a consistent service from one office to another, or even from one worker to another. There is no standard or guarantee of the service which an abused woman will receive—it may be excellent, mediocre or appalling. The reasons underlying this inconsistency can be found in the lack of training, knowledge of resources, policy statements and good practice guidelines" (1994:92).

3. Domestic Violence and the Role of General Practice

1. For a more extensive review of domestic violence research in the 1970s see Gelles (1980).

2. The Department of Health is Britain's governmental health authority. For further information see http://www.doh.gov.uk.

3. For example, Borkowski, Murch, and Walker (1983:24) report GPs' estimates of frequency of meeting cases of marital violence. The answers of the fifty GPs they interviewed ranged from once a week (2 percent), once a fortnight (9 percent), once a month (35 percent), once every three months (24 percent), once every six months (15 percent), once a year (11 percent), to less often (4 percent). Results from a postal survey in a Midlands county yielded similar results: out of 254 GPs, 15.5 percent stated that they saw women who are suspected of having experienced violence more than once a month, 76 percent said they encountered suspected victims only occasionally, and 8.5 percent claimed they had never seen any women who might be suffering abuse (Abbott and Williamson 1999:90).

4. A study of the economic implications of domestic violence estimated between 87,000 and 136,000 general practice consultations related to domestic violence per annum in Scotland (Young 1995). Statistical data from the United States reveal that "medical expenses arising from domestic violence assaults cost more than $44 million per year and result in 21,000 hospitalizations with 99,800 patient days of hospitalization, 28,700 emergency department visits, and 39,900 visits to physicians each year" (Schornstein 1997:4). We may assume that costs related to domestic violence could be even higher, considering the fact that a lot of women self-medicate or utilize friends, relatives, or informal health services (Williamson 2000). Costs for health care certainly also increase over time because of long-term chronic illness or mental health problems. More recently, the World Health Organization has also discussed the economic implications of interpersonal violence and has called for action (Khan 2004).

5. Grampian Health Board, which is now subsumed under the Grampian NHS Board, is the regional health authority whose main functions are strategic overview of the NHS

(National Health Service) in Grampian, including the allocation of Scottish Executive funding, public health, and health promotion.

6. I am not implying that practices in more deprived areas would have more patients suffering domestic violence, although doctors working in such areas seemed on the whole (although not all of them) to be more aware of the problem. However, this does not necessarily support the commonly held myth that domestic violence is also a social class issue. As some GPs pointed out, there may be more of a "hidden agenda" in the higher social classes (see chapter 5).

7. We must not forget, however, that transcriptions are merely symbolic representations of interviews, the recordings of which are primarily auditory in nature. This has implications for the validity of transcriptions, as Bailey, Maynor, and Cukor-Avila assert: "Only recordings themselves have validity as texts: transcriptions serve as a guide to the contents of the recordings and as an aid in auditing them. Transcriptions of recordings are not reproductions but interpretations of texts, and like all other interpretive acts they reflect the training, biases, and linguistic experiences of the transcriber" (1991:14).

8. To "have face," in Goffman's adoption of the Chinese concept, means that a person's pattern of verbal and nonverbal acts "presents an image of him that is internally consistent, that is supported by judgments and evidence conveyed by other participants, and that is confirmed by evidence conveyed through impersonal agencies in the situation" (1967:6–7). People attempt to portray themselves in as favorable a light as possible, and this attempt is usually mutual and therefore coconstructive.

5. Setting the Scene of Abuse

1. On the level of cognition and memory this shows that the retrieval of one narrative often triggers the remembrance of other related or similar stories. As Norrick (1998, 2000) points out, this process of "telling back" a similar story occurs frequently in everyday conversations, where conversationalists take turns in relating stories. In the 1960s Harvey Sacks called this phenomenon of telling a next story that parallels a previous one "second storying" and explained it as an indication of shared knowledge among speakers. Strictly speaking, this particular story is not a second but a serial story, since it is one of a set by the same speaker.

2. A more detailed overview of modalities and further examples are provided in chapter 7.

3. The term *vector* is used in Linde and Labov's (1975) study of people's descriptions of the layouts of their apartments to denote directions of movements. Linde and Labov found that there were direct links between cognitive input, discourse rules, and the rules of sentence grammar in people's descriptions.

4. Incidentally, medical doctors appear to be especially prone to employing war metaphors when describing their activities (Gwyn 1999:206). As Sontag (1991) argues, the

military metaphor is dangerous, as it provides an argument for marginalizing and repressing certain illnesses and patients.

5. It is important to note that patients likewise separate medical and private spheres, which, in the case of domestic violence issues, may also lead to women's reluctance to broach the problem with medical professionals.

6. Mythologizing Time, Mythologizing Violence

1. "Ach," sometimes transcribed as "och," is a Scottish locution equivalent to "oh, my."

7. Agents of Their Own Victimization

1. Whalen, Zimmerman, and Whalen (1988) observe a similarly routinized procedure in emergency service encounters. Calls to an emergency service number "exhibit, within a range of orderly variation, a distinctive organization of sequences as follows: (1) Opening/Identification, (2) Request, (2a) Interrogative Series, (3) Response, (4) Closing" (Whalen, Zimmerman, and Whalen 1988:342).

2. For an overview of various theories see Schornstein (1997:55–62).

3. Cornhill Hospital is the local psychiatric clinic.

8. Evaluating Abuse

1. The term *hedged performative* goes back to George Lakoff's (1972) article on hedges, in which he mentions the observation made by Robin Lakoff that certain syntactical constructions such as "I think/suppose/guess that . . ." express performatives that avoid commitment. Fraser applied this concept to the discussion of modal verbs and quasi modals.

9. Conclusion

1. The Zero Tolerance Charitable Trust is an independent charity that campaigns for the prevention of male violence against women and children. The trust was established in 1995 and works mainly in the United Kingdom and Europe.

2. A book that has already begun to compile suggestions for topics, texts, and methods in teaching literature to medical students is Hawkins and McEntyre's *Teaching Literature and Medicine* (2000).

Bibliography

Abbott, Pamela, and Emma Williamson. 1999. "Women, Health and Domestic Violence." *Journal of Gender Studies* 8.1:83–102.

Adam, Barbara. 1995. *Timewatch: The Social Analysis of Time.* Cambridge: Polity Press.

Ainsworth-Vaughn, Nancy. 1998. *Claiming Power in Doctor-Patient Talk.* Oxford: Oxford University Press.

Annandale, Ellen. 1998. *The Sociology of Health and Medicine: A Critical Introduction.* Cambridge: Polity Press.

Antaki, Charles, and Sue Widdicombe. 1998. "Identity as an Achievement and as a Tool." In Charles Antaki and Sue Widdicombe, eds., *Identities in Talk*, 1–14. London: Sage.

Auer, Peter, Elizabeth Couper-Kuhlen, and Frank Müller. 1999. *Language in Time: The Rhythm and Tempo of Spoken Interaction.* Oxford: Oxford University Press.

Bailey, Guy, Natalie Maynor, and Patricia Cukor-Avila. 1991. "Introduction." In Guy Bailey, Natalie Maynor, and Patricia Cukor-Avila, eds., *The Emergence of Black English: Text and Commentary*, 1–20. Amsterdam: John Benjamins.

Bamberg, Michael G. W., ed. 1997. "Oral Versions of Personal Experience: Three Decades of Narrative Analysis." Special issue of *Journal of Narrative and Life History* 7:1–415.

Barthes, Roland. 1972. *Mythologies.* Trans. Annette Lavers. London: Jonathan Cape.

Bennett, A. E., ed. 1976. *Communication between Doctors and Patients.* Oxford: Oxford University Press.

Birus, Hendrik. 2000. "Metapher." In Harald Fricke, ed., *Reallexikon der deutschen Literaturwissenschaft*, 2:571–76. Berlin: de Gruyter.

Boden, Deirdre, and Don H. Zimmerman, eds. 1991. *Talk and Social Structure: Studies in Ethnomethodology and Conversation Analysis.* Cambridge: Polity Press.

Bograd, Michele. 1987. "Battered Women, Cultural Myths and Clinical Interventions: A Feminist Analysis." *Women and Therapy* 5:69–77.

Borkowski, Margaret, Mervyn Murch, and Val Walker. 1983. *Marital Violence: The Community Response.* London: Tavistock.

Bourdieu, Pierre. 1991. *Language and Symbolic Power.* Ed. John B. Thompson. Trans. Gino Raymond and Matthew Adamson. Cambridge: Polity Press.

Bower, Anne R. 1997. "Deliberative Action Constructs: Reference and Evaluation in
    Narrative." In Guy et al. 1997:57–75.

Bradley, Fiona, et al. 2002. "Reported Frequency of Domestic Violence: Cross-
    Sectional Survey of Women Attending General Practice." *British Medical
    Journal* 324:271–73.

British Medical Association. 1998. *Domestic Violence: A Healthcare Issue?* London:
    BMA Board of Science and Education.

Brown, Gillian. 1995. *Speakers, Listeners and Communication: Explorations in
    Discourse Analysis.* Cambridge: Cambridge University Press.

Brown, Julie R., and L. Edna Rogers. 1991. "Openness, Uncertainty, and Intimacy: An
    Epistemological Reformulation." In Nikolas Coupland, Howard Giles, and
    John M. Wiemann, eds., *"Miscommunication" and Problematic Talk*, 146–
    65. Newbury Park: Sage.

Brown, Penelope, and Stephen C. Levinson. 1987. *Politeness: Some Universals in
    Language Usage.* Cambridge: Cambridge University Press.

Bruner, Jerome. 1986. *Actual Minds, Possible Worlds.* Cambridge MA: Harvard
    University Press.

———. 1991. "The Narrative Construction of Reality." *Critical Inquiry* 18:1–21.

———. 2003. *Making Stories: Law, Literature, Life.* Cambridge MA: Harvard
    University Press.

Bunch, Charlotte. 1997. "The Intolerable Status Quo: Violence against Women and
    Girls." In UNICEF, *The Progress of Nations*, 41–45. http://www.unicef.org/
    pon97/40–49.pdf. Accessed May 30, 2006.

Cameron, Lynne. 1999. "Operationalising 'Metaphor' for Applied Linguistic
    Research." In Cameron and Low 1999:3–28.

Cameron, Lynne, and Graham Low, eds. 1999. *Researching and Applying Metaphor.*
    Cambridge: Cambridge University Press.

Campbell, Jacquelyn C. 1992. "Ways of Teaching, Learning and Knowing about
    Violence against Women." *Nursing and Health Care* 13:464–70.

———. 2002. "Health Consequences of Intimate Partner Violence." *Lancet*
    359:1331–36.

Campbell, Jacquelyn C., et al. 1994. "Battered Women's Experiences in the Emergency
    Department." *Journal of Emergency Nursing* 20.4:280–88.

Celce-Murcia, Marianne, and Diane Larsen-Freeman. 1983. *The Grammar Book: An
    ESL/EFL Teacher's Course.* Rowley: Newbury House Publishers.

Celi, Ana, and Maria Christina Boiero. 2002. "The Heritage of Stories: A Tradition of
    Wisdom." *American Studies International* 40.2:57–72.

Charon, Rita. 2005. "Narrative Medicine: Attention, Representation, Affiliation."
    Narrative 13.3:261–70.

Chomsky, Noam. 1988. *Language and Problems of Knowledge: The Managua Lectures.*
    Cambridge MA: MIT Press.

Cicourel, Aaron V. 1981. "Language and Medicine." In Charles Ferguson et al., eds., *Language in the U.S.A.*, 407–29. Cambridge: Cambridge University Press.

Cohen, Sherrill. 1992. *The Evolution of Women's Asylums since 1500: From Refuges for Ex-Prostitutes to Shelters for Battered Women.* Oxford: Oxford University Press.

Coid, Jeremy, et al. 2001. "Relation between Childhood Sexual and Physical Abuse and Risk of Revictimisation in Women: A Cross-Sectional Survey." *Lancet* 358:450–54.

Couser, G. Thomas. 1997. *Recovering Bodies: Illness, Disability, and Life Writing.* Madison: University of Wisconsin Press.

Crossley, Michele L. 2000. *Introducing Narrative Psychology: Self, Trauma and the Construction of Meaning.* Buckingham: Open University Press.

Cushing, Steven. 1990. "Social/Cognitive Mismatch as a Source of Fatal Language Errors." Paper presented at the 1990 International Pragmatics Conference, Barcelona.

———. 1994. *Fatal Words: Communication Clashes and Aircraft Crashes.* Chicago: University of Chicago Press.

Daiute, Colette, and Katherine Nelson. 1997. "Making Sense of the Sense-Making Function of Narrative Evaluation." In Bamberg 1997:207–15.

De Fina, Anna, Deborah Schiffrin, and Michael Bamberg, eds. 2006. *Discourse and Identity.* Cambridge: Cambridge University Press.

Dell, Pippa, and Onkar Korotana. 2000. "Accounting for Domestic Violence: A Q Methodological Study." *Violence against Women* 6.3:286–310.

Dent-Read, Cathy C., and Agnes Szokolszky. 1993. "Where Do Metaphors Come From?" *Metaphor and Symbolic Activity* 8.3:227–42.

Department of Health, United Kingdom. 2000. *Domestic Violence: A Resource Manual for Health Care Professionals.* London: Department of Health.

de Rivera, Joseph, and Theodore R. Sarbin, eds. 1998. *Believed-In Imaginings: The Narrative Construction of Reality.* Washington DC: American Psychological Association.

Dingwall, Robert. 1992. "'Don't Mind Him—He's from Barcelona': Qualitative Methods in Health Studies." In Jeanne Daly, Ian McDonald, and Ewan Willis, eds., *Researching Health Care: Designs, Dilemmas, Disciplines*, 161–75. London: Routledge.

Dittmar, Norbert, and Ursula Bredel. 1999. *Die Sprachmauer: Die Verarbeitung der Wende und ihrer Folgen in Gesprächen mit Ost-und WestberlinerInnen.* Berlin: Weidler.

Dobash, R. Emerson, and Russell Dobash. 1979. *Violence against Wives: A Case against the Patriarchy.* London: Open Books.

Dobash, R. Emerson, Russell P. Dobash, and Katherine Cavanagh. 1985. "The Contact between Battered Women and Social and Medical Agencies." In Pahl 1985:142–65.

Donald, Anne. 1998. "The Words We Live In." In Greenhalgh and Hurwitz 1998:17–26.

Downie, Robert Silcock. 1991. "Literature and Medicine." *Journal of Medical Ethics* 17:93–96, 98.

Downs, Roger M., and David Stea. 1977. *Maps in Minds: Reflections on Cognitive Mapping.* New York: Harper and Row.

Eagleton, Terry. 1996. *Literary Theory: An Introduction.* 2nd ed. Oxford: Blackwell.

Eckert, Penelope, and Sally McConnell-Ginet. 1992. "Think Practically and Look Locally: Language and Gender as Community-Based Practice." *Annual Review of Anthropology* 21:461–90.

Eekelaar, John M., and Sanford N. Katz. 1978. *Family Violence: An International and Interdisciplinary Study.* Toronto: Butterworths.

Ehrlich, Susan. 1999. "Communities of Practice, Gender, and the Representation of Sexual Assault." *Language in Society* 28.2:239–56.

———. 2001. *Representing Rape: Language and Sexual Consent.* London: Routledge.

Elwyn, Glyn, and Richard Gwyn. 1998. "Stories we hear and stories we tell . . . Analysing Talk in Clinical Practice." In Greenhalgh and Hurwitz 1998:165–75.

Fairclough, Norman. 1989. *Language and Power.* London: Longman.

———. 1992. *Discourse and Social Change.* Cambridge: Polity Press.

———. 2001. *Language and Power.* 2nd ed. Harlow: Longman.

Farrell, Thomas B. 1985. "Narrative in Natural Discourse: On Conversation and Rhetoric." *Journal of Communication* 35.4:109–27.

Fasold, Ralph. 1990. *The Sociolinguistics of Language.* Oxford: Blackwell.

Fillmore, Charles J. 1968. "The Case for Case." In Emmon Bach and Robert T. Harms, eds., *Universals in Linguistic Theory,* 1–88. New York: Holt, Rinehart and Winston.

Fisher, Sue, and Alexandra Dundas Todd, eds. 1983. *The Social Organization of Doctor-Patient Communication.* Washington DC: Center for Applied Linguistics.

Fisher, Walter R. 1984. "Narration as a Human Communication Paradigm: The Case of Public Moral Argument." *Communication Monographs* 51:1–22.

———. 1985. "The Narrative Paradigm: In the Beginning." *Journal of Communication* 35.4:74–89.

Fludernik, Monika. 1996. *Towards a "Natural" Narratology.* London: Routledge.

Foucault, Michel. 1973. *The Birth of the Clinic.* Trans. A. M. Sheridan. London: Tavistock.

———. 1981. "The Order of Discourse." In Robert Young, ed., *Untying the Text: A Post-Structuralist Reader,* 48–78. Boston: Routledge and Kegan Paul.

———. 1982. "Afterword: The Subject and Power." In Hubert L. Dreyfus and Paul Rabinow, *Michel Foucault: Beyond Structuralism and Hermeneutics,* 208–26. New York: Harvester Wheatsheaf.

Frank, Arthur W. 1995. *The Wounded Storyteller: Body, Illness and Ethics*. Chicago: University of Chicago Press.

Fraser, Bruce. 1975. "Hedged Performatives." In Peter Cole and Jerry L. Morgan, eds., *Syntax and Semantics*, vol. 3: *Speech Acts*, 187–210. New York: Harcourt Brace and Jovanovich.

García-Moreno, C. 2002. "Dilemmas and Opportunities for an Appropriate Health-Service Response to Violence against Women." *Lancet* 359:1509–14.

Gay, William C. 1997. "The Reality of Linguistic Violence against Women." In Laura L. O'Toole and Jessica R. Schiffman, eds., *Gender Violence: Interdisciplinary Perspectives*, 467–73. New York: New York University Press.

Gelles, Richard J. 1976. "Abused Wives: Why Do They Stay?" *Journal of Marriage and the Family* 38:659–68.

———. 1980. "Violence in the Family: A Review of Research in the Seventies." *Journal of Marriage and the Family* 42:873–85.

Gibbs, Raymond W. 1999. "Researching Metaphor." In Cameron and Graham 1999:29–47.

Giles, Howard, and Robert N. St. Clair, eds. 1979. *Language and Social Psychology*. Oxford: Blackwell.

Giles, Howard, and Philip Smith. 1979. "Accommodation Theory: Optimal Levels of Convergence." In Giles and St. Clair 1979:45–65.

Glaser, Barney G., and Anselm L. Strauss. 1967. *The Discovery of Grounded Theory: Strategies for Qualitative Research*. Chicago: Aldine.

Goffman, Erving. 1967. *Interaction Ritual: Essays on Face-to-Face Behaviour*. London: Allen Lane.

———. 1974. *Frame Analysis*. Harmondsworth: Penguin.

Greenhalgh, Trisha, and Brian Hurwitz, eds. 1998. *Narrative Based Medicine: Dialogue and Discourse in Clinical Practice*. London: BMJ Books.

Grice, H. Paul. 1999 [1975]. "Logic and Conversation." In Jaworski and Coupland 1999:76–88.

Gruber, Jeffrey Steven. 1965. "Studies in Lexical Relations." Ph.D. dissertation, MIT, Cambridge MA.

Gumperz, John J. 1997. "On the Interactional Bases of Speech Community Membership." In Guy et al. 1997:183–203.

Gumperz, John J., and Jenny Cook-Gumperz. 1982. "Introduction: Language and the Communication of Social Identity." In John J. Gumperz, ed., *Language and Social Identity*, 1–21. Cambridge: Cambridge University Press.

Guy, Gregory, et al., eds. 1997. *Towards a Social Science of Language: Papers in Honour of William Labov*, vol. 2: *Social Interaction and Discourse Structures*. Amsterdam: John Benjamins.

Gwyn, Richard. 1999. "'Captain of my own ship': Metaphor and the Discourse of Chronic Illness." In Cameron and Low 1999:203–20.

Hague, Gill, and Claudia Wilson. 2000. "The Silenced Pain: Domestic Violence 1945–1970." *Journal of Gender Studies* 9.2:157–69.

Hague, Gill, et al. 2002. "Abused Women's Perspectives: The Responsiveness of Domestic Violence Provision and Inter-Agency Initiatives." VRP *Summary Findings*. http://www.1.rhul.ac.uk/sociopolitical-science/vrp/Findings/rfhague.pdf. Accessed May 30, 2006.

Haslam, S. Alexander, et al. 2002. "From Personal Pictures in the Head to Collective Tools in the World: How Shared Stereotypes Allow Groups to Represent and Change Social Reality." In McGarty, Yzerbyt, and Spears 2002:157–85.

Hawkins, Anne Hunsaker, and Marilyn Chandler McEntyre, eds. 2000. *Teaching Literature and Medicine*. New York: Modern Language Association of America.

Henderson, S. 1997. *Service Provision to Women Experiencing Domestic Violence in Scotland*. Edinburgh: Scottish Office Central Research Unit.

Herman, David. 1997. "Scripts, Sequences, and Stories: Elements of a Postclassical Narratology." PMLA 112.5:1046–59.

———, ed. 1999a. *Narratologies: New Perspectives on Narrative Analysis*. Columbus: Ohio State University Press.

———. 1999b. "Toward a Socionarratology: New Ways of Analyzing Natural-Language Narratives." In Herman 1999a:218–46.

———. 2001. "Spatial Reference in Narrative Domains." *Text* 21.4:515–41.

———. 2002. *Story Logic: Problems and Possibilities of Narrative*. Lincoln: University of Nebraska Press.

Hinnenkamp, Volker. 1998. *Mißverständnisse in Gesprächen: Eine empirische Untersuchung im Rahmen der Interpretativen Soziolinguistik*. Opladen: Westdeutscher Verlag.

Holmes, Janet. 1995. *Women, Men and Politeness*. London: Longman.

Home Office, United Kingdom. 2000. *Government Policy around Domestic Violence*. London: Home Office.

Hudson-Allez, Glyn. 1997. *Time-Limited Therapy in a General Practice Setting: How to Help within Six Sessions*. London: Sage.

Hunter, Kathryn Montgomery. 1991. *Doctors' Stories: The Narrative Structure of Medical Knowledge*. Princeton: Princeton University Press.

Hunter, Kathryn Montgomery, Rita Charon, and John L. Coulehan. 1995. "The Study of Literature in Medical Education." *Academic Medicine* 70.9:787–94.

Hydén, Lars-Christer. 1997. "Illness and Narrative." *Sociology of Health and Illness* 19.1:48–69.

Imbens-Bailey, Alison, and Allyssa McCabe. 2000. "The Discourse of Distress: A Narrative Analysis of Emergency Calls to 911." *Language and Communication* 20:275–96.

Jackendoff, Ray S. 1972. *Semantic Interpretation in Generative Grammar*. Cambridge MA: MIT Press.

———. 2002. *Foundations of Language: Brain, Meaning, Grammar, Evolution.* Oxford: Oxford University Press.

Jahn, Manfred. 1999. "'Speak, friend, and enter': Garden Paths, Artificial Intelligence, and Cognitive Narratology." In Herman 1999a:167–94.

Jaworski, Adam, and Nikolas Coupland, eds. 1999. *The Discourse Reader.* London: Routledge.

Johnson, Holly. 2001. "Contrasting Views of the Role of Alcohol in Cases of Wife Assault." *Journal of Interpersonal Violence* 16.1:54–72.

Johnson, Mark. 1987. *The Body in the Mind: The Bodily Basis of Meaning, Imagination, and Reason.* Chicago: University of Chicago Press.

Johnson, Michael P., and Kathleen J. Ferraro. 2000. "Research on Domestic Violence in the 1990s: Making Distinctions." *Journal of Marriage and the Family* 62:948–63.

Johnson, Norman. 1995. "Domestic Violence: An Overview." In Kingston and Penhale 1995:101–26.

Johnstone, Barbara. 1990. *Stories, Community and Place: Narratives from Middle America.* Bloomington: Indiana University Press.

Jonsen, Albert R. 2000. *A Short History of Medical Ethics.* Oxford: Oxford University Press.

Kanyó, Zoltán. 1986. "Narrative and Communication: An Attempt to Formulate Some Principles for a Theoretical Account of Narrative." *Neohelicon* 13.2:107–31.

Keller, L. Eileen. 1996. "Invisible Victims: Battered Women in Psychiatric and Medical Emergency Rooms." *Bulletin of the Menninger Clinic* 60.1:1–21.

Khan, Abdullah. 2004. "WHO Argues the Economic Case for Tackling Violence." *Lancet* 363:2058.

Kingston, Paul, and Bridget Penhale, eds. 1995. *Family Violence and the Caring Professions.* Basingstoke: Macmillan.

Kirmayer, Laurence J. 2000. "Broken Narratives: Clinical Encounters and the Poetics of Illness Experience." In Mattingly and Garro 2000:153–80.

Kurz, Demie, and Evan Stark. 1990. "Not-So-Benign Neglect: The Medical Response to Battering." In Yl10 and Bograd 1990:249–66.

Labov, William. 1972a. *Language in the Inner City: Studies in the Black English Vernacular.* Philadelphia: University of Pennsylvania Press.

———. 1972b. *Sociolinguistic Patterns.* Philadelphia: University of Pennsylvania Press.

———. 1982. "Speech Actions and Reactions in Personal Narrative." In Tannen 1982:219–47.

———. 1997. "Some Further Steps in Narrative Analysis." In Bamberg 1997:396–415.

Labov, William, and Joshua Waletzky. 1967. "Narrative Analysis: Oral Versions of Personal Experience." In June Helm, ed., *Essays on the Verbal and Visual Arts,* 12–44. Seattle: University of Washington Press.

Labov, William, and Wendell A. Harris. 1994. "Addressing Social Issues through
    Linguistic Evidence." In John Gibbons, ed., *Language and the Law*, 265–305.
    London: Longman.
LaFrance, Marianne, and Eugene Hahn. 1994. "The Disappearing Agent: Gender
    Stereotypes, Interpersonal Verbs, and Implicit Causality." In Camille
    Roman, Suzanne Juhasz, and Cristanne Miller, eds., *The Woman and
    Language Debate: A Sourcebook*, 348–62. New Brunswick: Rutgers
    University.
Laing, Ronald D., Herbert Phillipson, and A. Russell Lee. 1966. *Interpersonal
    Perception: A Theory and a Method of Research*. London: Tavistock.
Lakoff, George. 1972. "Hedges: A Study of Meaning Criteria and the Logic of Fuzzy
    Concepts." In P. Peranteau, J. Levi, and G. Phares, eds., *Papers from the
    Eighth Regional Meeting of the Chicago Linguistic Society*, 183–228. Chicago:
    University of Chicago Press.
———. 1993. "The Contemporary Theory of Metaphor." In Ortony 1993:202–51.
Lakoff, George, and Mark Johnson. 1980. *Metaphors We Live By*. Chicago: University
    of Chicago Press.
Lakoff, Robin. 1977. "What You Can Do with Words: Politeness, Pragmatics and
    Performatives." In Andy Rogers, Bob Wall, and John Murphy, eds.,
    *Proceedings of the Texas Conference on Performatives, Presuppositions and
    Implicatures*, 79–106. Arlington: Center for Applied Linguistics.
Lamb, Sharon. 1999. "Constructing the Victim: Popular Images and Lasting Labels."
    In Sharon Lamb, ed., *New Versions of Victims: Feminists Struggle with the
    Concept*, 108–38. New York: New York University Press.
Langellier, Kristin M., and Eric E. Peterson. 2004. *Storytelling in Daily Life:
    Performing Narrative*. Philadelphia: Temple University Press.
Lanser, Susan S. 1981. *The Narrative Act: Point of View in Prose Fiction*. Princeton:
    Princeton University Press.
Laurier, Eric. 1999. "Talking about Cigarettes: Conversational Narratives about
    Health and Illness." *Health* 3.2:189–207.
Lawless, Elaine. 2001. *Women Escaping Violence: Empowerment through Narrative*.
    Columbia: University of Missouri Press.
Leech, Geoffrey N. 1987. *Meaning and the English Verb*. 2nd ed. London: Longman.
Lévi-Strauss, Claude. 1986. "The Structural Study of Myth." In Hazard Adams and
    Leroy Searle, eds., *Critical Theory since 1965*, 809–22. Tallahassee: Florida
    State University Press.
Lind, E. Allan, and William M. O'Barr. 1979. "The Social Significance of Speech in
    the Courtroom." In Giles and St. Clair 1979:66–87.
Linde, Charlotte. 1997a. "Discourse Analysis, Structuralism, and the Description of
    Social Practice." In Guy et al. 1997:3–29.
———. 1997b. "Narrative: Experience, Memory, Folklore." In Bamberg 1997:281–89.

————. 1999. "The Transformation of Narrative Syntax into Institutional Memory." *Narrative Inquiry* 9.1:139–74.

Linde, Charlotte, and William Labov. 1975. "Spatial Networks as a Site for the Study of Language and Thought." *Language* 51.4:924–39.

Lloyd, Siobhan. 1995. "Social Work and Domestic Violence." In Kingston and Penhale 1995:149–77.

Loseke, Donileen R., and Spencer E. Cahill. 1984. "The Social Construction of Deviance: Experts on Battered Women." *Social Problems* 31.3:296–310.

Marková, Ivana, and Klaus Foppa. 1991. "Conclusion." In Ivana Marková and Klaus Foppa, eds., *Asymmetries in Dialogue*, 259–73. Hemel Hempstead: Harvester Wheatsheaf.

Mason, Jennifer. 1996. *Qualitative Researching*. London: Sage.

Mattingly, Cheryl. 2000. "Emergent Narratives." In Mattingly and Garro 2000:181–211.

Mattingly, Cheryl, and Linda C. Garro, eds. 2000. *Narrative and the Cultural Construction of Illness and Healing*. Berkeley: University of California Press.

Maynard, Douglas W. 1988. "Language, Interaction, and Social Problems." *Social Problems* 35.4:311–34.

Mazza, Danielle, Lorraine Dennerstein, and Vicky Ryan. 1996. "Physical, Sexual and Emotional Violence against Women: A General Practice-Based Prevalence Study." *Medical Journal of Australia* 164:14–17.

McGarty, Craig. 2002. "Stereotype Formation as Category Formation." In McGarty, Yzerbyt, and Spears 2002:16–37.

McGarty, Craig, Russell Spears, and Vincent Y. Yzerbyt. 2002. "Conclusion: Stereotypes Are Selective, Variable and Contested Explanations." In McGarty, Yzerbyt, and Spears 2002:186–99.

McGarty, Craig, Vincent Y. Yzerbyt, and Russell Spears, eds. 2002. *Stereotypes as Explanations: The Formation of Meaningful Beliefs about Social Groups*. Cambridge: Cambridge University Press.

McKie, Linda. 2004. *Families, Violence and Social Change*. Buckingham: Open University Press.

McKie, Linda, Barbara Fennell, and Jarmila Mildorf. 2002. "Time to Disclose, Timing Disclosure: GPs' Discourses on Disclosing Domestic Abuse in Primary Care." *Sociology of Health and Illness* 24.3:327–46.

McLellan, M. Faith. 1997. "Literature and Medicine: Narratives of Physical Illness." *Lancet* 349:1618–20.

Meredith, Philip. 1993. "Patient Participation in Decision-Making and Consent to Treatment: The Case of General Surgery." *Sociology of Health and Illness* 15.3:315–36.

Meyers, Marian. 1997. *News Coverage of Violence against Women: Engendering Blame*. Thousand Oaks: Sage.

Mezey, Gill, et al. 2002. "An Exploration of the Prevalence, Nature and Effects of Domestic Violence in Pregnancy." *VRP Summary Findings*. http://www1. rhul.ac.uk/sociopolitical-science/vrp/Findings/rfmezey.pdf. Accessed May 30, 2006.

Mildorf, Jarmila. 2002. "'Opening up a Can of Worms': Physicians' Narrative Construction of Knowledge about Domestic Violence." *Narrative Inquiry* 12.2:233–60.

———. 2004. "Narratives of Domestic Violence Cases: GPs Defining Their Professional Role." In Peter L. Twohig and Vera Kalitzkus, eds., *Making Sense of Health, Illness and Disease*, 177–200. Amsterdam: Rodopi.

Mishler, Elliot G. 1984. *The Discourse of Medicine: Dialectics of Medical Interviews*. Norwood: Ablex.

Mooney, Jayne. 2000. *Gender, Violence and the Social Order*. Basingstoke: Macmillan.

Norrick, Neal R. 1998. "Retelling Stories in Spontaneous Conversation." *Discourse Processes* 25.1:75–97.

———. 2000. *Conversational Narrative: Storytelling in Everyday Talk*. Amsterdam: John Benjamins.

Nünning, Ansgar, and Vera Nünning, eds. 2002a. *Erzähltheorie transgenerisch, intermedial, interdisziplinär*. Trier: Wissenschaftlicher Verlag Trier.

———, eds. 2002b. *Neue Ansätze in der Erzähltheorie*. Trier: Wissenschaftlicher Verlag Trier.

O'Connor, Bonnie Blair. 1995. *Healing Traditions: Alternative Medicine and the Health Professions*. Philadelphia: University of Pennsylvania Press.

Ortony, Andrew, ed. 1993. *Metaphor and Thought*. 2nd ed. Cambridge: Cambridge University Press.

Pahl, Jan. ed. 1985. *Private Violence and Public Policy: The Needs of Battered Women and the Response of the Public Services*. London: Routledge and Kegan Paul.

———. 1995. "Health Professionals and Violence against Women." In Kingston and Penhale 1995:127–48.

Perkins, Jane M., and Nancy Blyler. 1999. "Introduction: Taking a Narrative Turn in Professional Communication." In Jane M. Perkins and Nancy Blyler, eds., *Narrative and Professional Communication*, 1–34. Stamford: Ablex.

Pinker, Steven. 1994. *The Language Instinct*. Harmondsworth: Penguin.

———. 1997. *How the Mind Works*. Harmondsworth: Penguin.

Polkinghorne, Donald E. 1995. "Narrative Configuration in Qualitative Analysis." In J. Amos Hatch et al., eds., *Life History and Narrative*, 2–23. London: Falmer.

Prickett, Stephen. 2002. *Narrative, Religion and Science: Fundamentalism versus Irony, 1700–1999*. Cambridge: Cambridge University Press.

Prince, Gerald. 1997. "Narratology and Narratological Analysis." In Bamberg 1997:39–44.

Propp, Vladimir. 1968. *Morphology of the Folktale*. 2nd ed. Trans. Laurence Scott; rev. Louis A. Wagner. Austin: University of Texas Press.

Ptacek, James. 1990. "Why Do Men Batter Their Wives?" In Yllö and Bograd
    1990:133–57.
Quirk, Randolph, et al. 1985. *A Comprehensive Grammar of the English Language.*
    London: Longman.
Rachman, Stephen. 1998. "Literature in Medicine." In Greenhalgh and Hurwitz
    1998:123–27.
Radford, Andrew. 1988. *Transformational Grammar: A First Course.* Cambridge:
    Cambridge University Press.
Radford, Jill, Melissa Friedberg, and Lynne Harne, eds. 2000. *Women, Violence and
    Strategies for Action: Feminist Research, Policy and Practice.* Buckingham:
    Open University Press.
Richardson, Jo, et al. 2001. "Women Who Experience Domestic Violence and Women
    Survivors of Childhood Sexual Abuse: A Survey of Health Professionals'
    Attitudes and Clinical Practice." *British Journal of General Practice*
    51:468–70.
———, et al. 2002. "Identifying Domestic Violence: Cross-Sectional Study in
    Primary Care." *British Medical Journal* 324:274.
Riessman, Catherine Kohler. 1993. *Narrative Analysis.* Newbury Park: Sage.
Rigney, Ann. 1992. "The Point of Stories: On Narrative Communication and Its
    Cognitive Functions." *Poetics Today* 13.2:263–83.
Robinson, John A., and Linda Hawpe. 1986. "Narrative Thinking as a Heuristic
    Process." In Theodore R. Sarbin, ed., *Narrative Psychology: The Storied
    Nature of Human Conduct,* 111–25. New York: Praeger.
Rosewater, Lynne Bravo. 1990. "Battered or Schizophrenic? Psychological Tests Can't
    Tell." In Yllö and Bograd 1990:200–216.
Rubin, Herbert, and Irene Rubin. 1995. *Qualitative Interviewing: The Art of Hearing
    Data.* London: Sage.
Sacks, Harvey, Emanuel A. Schegloff, and Gail Jefferson. 1974. "A Simplest
    Systematics for the Organization of Turn-Taking for Conversation."
    Language 50.4:696–735.
Sanders, Robert E. 2005. "Validating 'Observations' in Discourse Studies: A
    Methodological Reason for Attention to Cognition." In te Molder and
    Potter 2005:57–78.
Sapir, Edward. 1949. "The Status of Linguistics as a Science." In David G.
    Mandelbaum, ed., *Selected Writings of Edward Sapir in Language, Culture
    and Personality,* 160–66. Berkeley: University of California Press.
Sarbin, Theodore R. 1986. "The Narrative as a Root Metaphor for Psychology." In
    Theodore R. Sarbin, ed., *Narrative Psychology: The Storied Nature of Human
    Conduct,* 3–21. New York: Praeger.
Schank, Roger C. 1990. *Tell Me a Story: Narrative and Intelligence.* Evanston:
    Northwestern University Press.

Schank, Roger C., and Robert P. Abelson. 1977. *Scripts, Plans, Goals and Understanding: An Inquiry into Human Knowledge Structures.* Hillsdale: Lawrence Erlbaum.

Schegloff, Emanuel A. 1997. "'Narrative Analysis' Thirty Years Later." In Bamberg 1997:97–106.

Schiffrin, Deborah. 1987. *Discourse Markers.* Cambridge: Cambridge University Press.

———. 1993. "'Speaking for Another' in Sociolinguistic Interviews: Alignments, Identities, and Frames." In Tannen 1993a:231–63.

———. 1996. "Narrative as Self-Portrait: Sociolinguistic Constructions of Identity." *Language in Society* 25.2:167–203.

Schornstein, Sherri L. 1997. *Domestic Violence and Health Care: What Every Professional Needs to Know.* Thousand Oaks: Sage.

Schütze, Fritz. 1981. "Prozeßstrukturen des Lebensablaufs." In Joachim Matthes, Arno Pfeifenberger, and Manfred Stosberg, eds., *Biographie in handlungswissenschaftlicher Perspektive,* 67–156. Nürnberg: Verlag der Nürnberger Forschungsvereinigung.

———. 1983. "Biographieforschung und narratives Interview." *Neue Praxis* 3:283–93.

Scott, Marvin B., and Stanford M. Lyman. 1968. "Accounts." *American Sociological Review* 33:46–62.

Scottish Executive. 2000. *National Strategy to Address Domestic Abuse in Scotland.* Edinburgh: Stationery Office.

———. 2001. *Preventing Violence against Women: Action across the Scottish Executive.* Edinburgh: Stationery Office.

Scottish Needs Assessment Programme. 1997. *Domestic Violence.* Glasgow: Scottish Forum for Public Health Medicine.

Scottish Parliament. 2000. *Domestic Abuse in Scotland.* Research Note RN 00/101. Edinburgh: Scottish Parliament.

———. 2001. *The Protection from Abuse (Scotland) Bill.* Research Note RN 01/65. Edinburgh: Scottish Parliament.

Shuy, Roger W. 1976. "The Medical Interview: Problems in Communication." *Primary Care* 3:365–86.

———. 1993. *Language Crimes: The Use and Abuse of Language Evidence in the Courtroom.* Oxford: Blackwell.

Silverman, David. 1987. *Communication and Medical Practice: Social Relations in the Clinic.* London: Sage.

Sontag, Susan. 1991. *Illness as Metaphor: AIDS and Its Metaphors.* London: Penguin.

Spears, Russell. 2002. "Four Degrees of Stereotype Formation: Differentiation by Any Means Necessary." In McGarty, Yzerbyt, and Spears 2002:127–56.

Spence, Donald P. 1998. "The Mythic Properties of Popular Explanations." In de Rivera and Sarbin 1998:217–28.

Squier, Harriet A. 1998. "Teaching Humanities in the Undergraduate Medical Curriculum." In Greenhalgh and Hurwitz 1998:128–39.

Stanko, Elizabeth A. 1985. *Intimate Intrusions: Women's Experience of Male Violence.* London: Routledge and Kegan Paul.

———. 1990. "Fear of Crime and the Myth of the Safe Home: A Feminist Critique of Criminology." In Yllö and Bograd 1990:75–88.

Steinmetz, Suzanne K., and Murray A. Straus. 1974. *Violence in the Family.* New York: Harper and Row.

Stern, Josef. 2000. *Metaphor in Context.* Cambridge MA: MIT Press.

Strong, Phil M. 1979. *The Ceremonial Order of the Clinic.* London: Routledge and Kegan Paul.

Sugg, Nancy Kathleen, and Thomas Inui. 1992. "Primary Care Physicians' Response to Domestic Violence: Opening Pandora's Box." *Journal of the American Medical Association* 267.23:3157–60.

Tannen, Deborah, ed. 1982. *Analyzing Discourse: Text and Talk.* Washington DC: Georgetown University Press.

———. 1989. *Talking Voices: Repetition, Dialogue, and Imagery in Conversational Discourse.* Cambridge: Cambridge University Press.

———, ed. 1993a. *Framing in Discourse.* Oxford: Oxford University Press.

———. 1993b. "What's in a Frame? Surface Evidence for Underlying Expectations." In Tannen 1993a:14–56.

Tannen, Deborah, and Cynthia Wallat. 1986. "Medical Professional and Parents: A Linguistic Analysis of Communication across Contexts." *Language in Society* 15:295–312.

Tayside Women and Violence Group. 1994. *Hit or Miss: An Exploratory Study of the Provision for Women Subjected to Domestic Violence in Tayside Region.* Tayside: Regional Council.

te Molder, Hedwig, and Jonathan Potter, eds. 2005. *Conversation and Cognition.* Cambridge: Cambridge University Press.

Tiersma, Peter, and Lawrence M. Solan. 2002. "The Linguist on the Witness Stand: Forensic Linguistics in American Courts." *Language* 78.2:221–39.

Titscher, Stefan, et al. 2000. *Methods of Text and Discourse Analysis.* Trans. Bryan Jenner. London: Sage.

Tolliver, Joyce. 1997. "From Labov and Waletzky to 'Contextualist Narratology': 1967–1997." In Bamberg 1997:53–60.

Toolan, Michael. 2001. *Narrative: A Critical Linguistic Introduction.* 2nd ed. London: Routledge.

Trinch, Shonna. 2001a. "The Advocate as Gatekeeper: The Limits of Politeness in Protective Order Interviews with Latina Survivors of Domestic Abuse." *Journal of Sociolinguistics* 5.4:475–506.

———. 2001b. "Managing Euphemism and Transcending Taboos: Negotiating the Meaning of Sexual Assault in Latinas' Narratives of Domestic Violence." *Text* 21.4:567–610.

————. 2003. *Latinas' Narratives of Domestic Abuse: Discrepant Versions of Violence.*
Amsterdam: John Benjamins.

Turner, Terence. 1991. "'We Are Parrots,' 'Twins Are Birds': Play of Tropes as
Operational Structure." In James W. Fernandez, ed., *Beyond Metaphor:
The Theory of Tropes in Anthropology*, 123–30. Stanford: Stanford University
Press.

Ulatowska, Hanna K., and Gloria Streit Olness. 1997. "Some Observations by Aphasics
and Their Contributions to Narrative Theory." In Bamberg 1997:259–64.

van Dijk, Teun A. 1997. "Discourse as Interaction in Society." In Teun A. van Dijk, ed.,
Discourse as Social Interaction, 1–37. London: Sage.

Wales, Katie. 2001. *A Dictionary of Stylistics.* 2nd ed. Harlow: Longman.

Warshaw, Carole. 1993. "Limitations of the Medical Model in the Care of Battered
Women." In Pauline B. Bart and Eileen Geil Moran, eds., *Violence against
Women: The Bloody Footprints*, 134–46. Newbury Park: Sage.

Wellberry, D. E. 1997. "Retrait/re-entry: Zur poststrukturalistischen
Metapherndiskussion." In Gerhard Neumann, ed., *Poststrukturalismus:
Herausforderung an die Literaturwissenschaft*, 194–207. Stuttgart: Metzler.

West, Candace. 1984. "Medical Misfires: Mishearings, Misgivings and
Misunderstandings in Physician-Patient Dialogues." *Discourse Processes*
7:107–34.

Whalen, Jack, Don H. Zimmerman, and Marylin R. Whalen. 1988. "When Words
Fail: A Single Case Analysis." *Social Problems* 35.4:335–62.

Williamson, Emma. 2000. *Domestic Violence and Health: The Response of the Medical
Profession.* Bristol: Policy Press.

Willson, Pam, et al. 2000. "Severity of Violence against Women by Intimate Partners
and Associated Use of Alcohol and/or Illicit Drugs by the Perpetrator."
Journal of Interpersonal Violence 15.9:996–1008.

Wilson, Thomas P. 1991. "Social Structure and the Sequential Organization of
Interaction." In Boden and Zimmerman 1991:22–43.

Wodak, Ruth. 1997. "Critical Discourse Analysis and the Study of Doctor-Patient
Interaction." In Britt-Louise Gunnarson, Per Linell, and Bengt Nordberg,
eds., *Construction of Professional Discourse*, 173–200. London: Longman.

Wolfson, Nessa. 1976. "Speech Events and Natural Speech: Some Implications for
Sociolinguistic Methodology." *Language in Society* 5.2:189–209.

Yllö, Kersti, and Michele Bograd, eds. 1990. *Feminist Perspectives on Wife Abuse.*
Newbury Park: Sage.

Young, D. 1995. "The Economic Implications of Domestic Violence in Greater
Glasgow." Master's thesis, University of York.

Young, Katharine. 1997. *Presence in the Flesh: The Body in Medicine.* Cambridge MA:
Harvard University Press.

Zimmerman, Don H., and Deirdre Boden. 1991. "Structure-in-Action: An
Introduction." In Boden and Zimmerman 1991:3–21.

Index

Abbott, Pamela, 31, 215n3
Abelson, Robert P., 20
Aberdeen, x, 36–37
abstract, 40
accommodation of speech, 6, 11, 41, 77, 107
accommodation theory, 45
action schemas, 58
active construction, 83, 127, 131. *See also* passive construction
actors, 7, 81, 114, 119, 125, 164
Adam, Barbara, 72
aesthetic approach, 183, 185
affective meaning, 4, 54
age, 6, 106
agency, 123, 124, 127, 151, 167; doctors', 7, 121, 140–43, 176; women's, 7, 34, 128–40, 159, 177
agens, 127–28, 135. See also *patiens*
Ainsworth-Vaughn, Nancy, 17, 126, 181
alcohol, 29, 106–7, 108–9, 132, 134, 139, 154, 157, 171, 175
Annandale, Ellen, 31, 33, 78, 112
Antaki, Charles, 17
anthropology, 10, 49
anxiety, 88–93, 176
artificial intelligence, 20
Auer, Peter, 162
authority, 87

back channels, 40, 43, 46, 48
backgrounds, 7, 37, 84, 89, 106–10, 111, 157, 160. *See also* alcohol; family history account; social class; sociodemographic factors
Bailey, Guy, 216n7
Bamberg, Michael, 13, 18
Barthes, Roland, 94, 102
battered women's movement, 28
Bennett, A. E., 25
biomedical model, 33–34, 78, 114, 115, 126, 143,

175, 176, 184
Birus, Hendrik, 68
blaming the victim, 104–5, 111, 136, 140, 177
Blyler, Nancy, 25
Boden, Deirdre, 213n3
Bograd, Michele, 27, 35, 139, 167
Boiero, Maria Christina, 3, 10, 68
Borkowski, Margaret, 27, 215n3
Bourdieu, Pierre, 3, 16, 102, 124
Bower, Ann, 149
Bradley, Fiona, 27, 214n9
Bredel, Ursula, 3, 12
British Medical Association, 30, 179
Brown, Gillian, 82
Brown, Julie R., 98–99
Brown, Penelope, 5, 46, 161
Bruner, Jerome, 4, 18–19, 39, 124, 154, 214n7
Bunch, Charlotte, ix
bureaucratic role format, 87, 117

Cahill, Spencer E., 22–23, 123, 140
Cameron, Lynne, 70
Campbell, Jacqueline, 27, 30, 181–82
case stories, 4, 23, 24
Cavanagh, Katherine, 27
Celce-Murcia, Marianne, 151
Celi, Ana, 3, 10, 68
ceremonial order, 17, 88, 125–26, 178
Charon, Rita, 182–83, 184
choice, 131, 133, 137–38, 142
Chomsky, Noam, 14
Cicourel, Aaron, 25
cliché, 75, 108, 110, 154, 167, 169, 179. *See also* stereotypes
coconstruction of narratives, 5, 42
coda, 40
code of practice, 45
cognition, 3, 19–20, 114

cognitive framework, 110
cognitive mapping, 71, 80, 88
cognitive maps, 71, 110–11
cognitive processes, 4, 19–20
Cohen, Sherrill, 28
Coid, Jeremy, 214n9
communication problems, 12, 32. *See also* miscommunication
community of practice, 25–26, 174–75
community response, 27
comparators, 76, 148, 151
complicating action, 12, 40
conceptual dependency theory, 20
confidentiality, 129
connectors, 98, 132, 135, 149, 156, 160, 161
constructed dialogue, 96, 108, 156–57, 175. *See also* direct speech
construction of reality, 3, 26, 105
consultation, 17, 22, 57, 59, 77, 99, 125, 157
consultation room, 73, 81
container metaphor, 82, 92, 113
context, 5, 11, 173. *See also* interview, situation
control, 92, 102
convergence, 45
Cook-Gumperz, Jenny, 27
corpus, 38–39. *See also* sample narratives
costs, 32, 215n4
Coulehan, John L., 182–83
countertransference, 35
Couper-Kuhlen, Elizabeth, 162
Couser, G. Thomas, 117
Critical Discourse Analysis, 3, 16
cross-domain mapping, 69. *See also* metaphor
Crossley, Michele, 17
Cukor-Avila, Patricia, 216n7
Cushing, Steven, 213n2
cycle-of-abuse theories, 29–30

Daiute, Colette, 146
data collection, 38–39. *See also* research methodology
defensiveness, 46, 77, 112
DeFina, Anna, 17
deliberative action construct, 149, 152
Dell, Pippa, 214n9
Dennerstein, Lorraine, 30, 31
Dent-Read, Cathy C., 68
Department of Health, 30–31, 179, 215n2
detachment, 170

deviance, 22, 65, 138–39, 156, 158, 161, 164, 166, 170, 176–77, 178. *See also* stigmatization
diagnosis, 17, 23
dialogue, 5, 44
diamond diagram of narratives, 5, 40, 64
Dingwall, Robert, 21
direct speech, 1, 54, 96, 108, 175. *See also* constructed dialogue
disclosure, 31, 50, 52–54, 67, 86, 98–99, 180
discourse, 3, 6, 8; as commodity, 3, 16, 102–3, 124; and knowledge, 3, 8; and power, 3, 14, 16–17, 94; scientific, 25. *See also* medical discourse
discourse markers, 119, 120, 132, 161
discursive psychology, 19
discursive strategies, 2, 152, 170
distancing, 81, 111, 132, 141, 177
Dittmar, Norbert, 3, 12
divergence, 45
Dobash, Emerson, 27, 28, 31
Dobash, Rebecca, 27, 28, 31
doctor-patient communication, 17, 21, 25, 32, 44, 95, 98
doctor-patient divide, 17, 133–34, 142–43, 177, 217n5
doctor-patient interaction, 22, 23, 33, 58–59
doctors' stories, 21–27. *See also* narrative, and medicine; patients' stories
domestic violence, 8, 30–33; and general practice, 27, 30–34; and illness, 30, 126, 215n4; political dimension of, 15, 28; prevalence of, ix; research, 28–29, 214n9
Donald, Anne, 17, 133–34, 177
Downie, Robert Silcock, 183
Downs, Roger M., 71
dramatism, 14–15
dramatization, 107, 154, 156–57, 159

Eagleton, Terry, 10
Eckert, Penelope, 25, 174
Eekelaar, John M., 27, 28
Ehrlich, Susan, 137–38
Elwyn, Glyn, 25
emergency calls, 12
empathic approach, 183, 185
ethical approach, 183, 185
ethnicity, 162
euphemism, 163, 214–15n10
evaluation, 7, 131, 144–46; and storied knowledge, 146–57, 171

excuses, 104, 109, 111, 176
expectations, 5, 42, 57–58, 87
expert knowledge, 17, 25, 112, 170, 179
explanations of domestic violence, 7, 29–30, 103–6, 107, 109, 138, 158, 175
explanatory models, 29

face-threatening acts, 46–47
face wants, 6, 113, 161
face work, 46, 114, 216n8
Fairclough, Norman, 3, 16, 23, 94, 175
family history account, 109, 157, 159, 175
Farrell, Thomas B., 13
Fasold, Ralph, 213n1
female-on-male violence, 164–72
feminist research, 6, 8, 29, 35
Fennell, Barbara, 99
Ferraro, Kathleen J., 29–30, 214n9
Fillmore, Charles J., 124, 127
Fisher, Sue, 25
Fisher, Walter, 14, 18
Fludernik, Monika, 13
folk knowledge, 25
folk language, 26, 83, 170, 179
Foppa, Klaus, 44
forensic linguistics, 213n2
Foucault, Michel, 3, 8, 21, 33, 73, 178
fragmentary narrative, 64, 214n6
frame, 41
frame, medical, 40
frame model, 5, 41–47
frames of expectation, 22, 79, 208
frame theory, 14, 41, 125
frameworks, social and natural, 125, 126, 127, 138, 140
Frank, Arthur, 58
Fraser, Bruce, 163, 217n1
frequency, 83–84, 215n3. *See also* presentation
Friedberg, Melissa, 214n9
frustration, 1, 32, 126

gaps, 167–68
García-Moreno, C., 181
gatekeeping, 24, 32–33, 37, 50
Gay, William C., 30
gaze, 73; deciphering, 73, 117; medical, 73, 178–79
Gelles, Richard J., 28, 29–30, 214n9, 215n1
gender, 6, 99, 129, 133, 139, 153–54, 164, 166–67

gerund, 129
Gibbs, Raymond, 73
Giles, Howard, 6, 45
Glaser, Barney, 58
Goffman, Erving: and face work, 6, 46, 113, 114, 216n8; and frame theory, 14, 41, 124, 125, 138
Grampian NHS Board, 37, 215–16n5
Greenhalgh, Trisha, 25
Grice, H. Paul, 5
Gricean maxims, 5
group: professional, 26, 117, 170; social, 15, 25. *See also* professionalism; roles
Gruber, Jeffrey Steven, 124, 127
Gumperz, John J., 27, 42
Gwyn, Richard, 25, 216n4

Hague, Gillian, 214n9
Hahn, Eugene, 158
Harne, Lynne, 214n9
Harris, Wendell A., 213n2
Haslam, S. Alexander, 9
Hawkins, Anne Hunsaker, 217n2
Hawpe, Linda, 12, 39
health services, 27, 31, 99
hedged performative, 163, 217n1
hedges, 46, 76, 113, 155, 156, 161–62, 214n6
helplessness. *See* powerlessness
Henderson, S., 31
Herman, David, 3, 71, 178, 214n5; and socionarratology, 3, 13–14, 131; and story logic, 3, 10–11, 39
Hinnenkamp, Volker, 213n2
Holmes, Janet, 46
Homo narrans, 14–15
Hudson-Allez, Glyn, 98
humor, 156, 166
Hunter, Kathryn Montgomery, 23, 24, 182–83
Hurwitz, Brian, 25
Hydén, Lars-Christer, 103

identity, 17–18, 47–48
ideology, 104–5
illness narratives, 58
Imbens-Bailey, Alison, 3, 5, 12
inadequacy, 32. *See also* myth, of inadequacy; powerlessness
inferences, 42

institutional memory, 26, 175, 176, 214n8, 215n10
institutions: and discourse, 16–17, 24, 26; and domestic violence, 28, 30
interaction, 3, 11, 19, 46. *See also* doctor-patient interaction
interpersonal perception, 45, 114, 121, 131
interpretation: of data, 8, 20, 49; in medicine, 23, 182
interview: format, 5; schedule, 38; situation, 41, 145; talk, 43
interviewee, 44–45
interviewer, 44–45
interviewer-initiated narratives, 39, 146. *See also* spontaneous narratives
interview frame, 5, 41, 44–47, 132, 148
interview narratives, 41–42
Inui, Thomas, 32, 95
involvement, 48, 119, 152, 156

Jackendoff, Ray, 114, 124, 127
Jahn, Manfred, 214n5
Jefferson, Gail, 44, 46
Johnson, Holly, 29, 108, 171, 214n9
Johnson, Mark, 69–70, 78–79, 82, 169
Johnson, Michael, 29–30
Johnson, Norman, 28, 29
Johnstone, Barbara, 17
Jonsen, Albert R., 127
journey metaphor, 88–89, 178
justifications, 104, 111, 176

Kanyó, Zoltán, 13
Katz, Sanford N., 27, 28
Keller, L. Eileen, 27, 35, 177
Khan, Abdullah, 215n4
Kirmayer, Laurence J., 10, 69, 70–71
knowledge: cultural, 3; of domestic violence, 2, 4, 8, 52, 66, 75, 153; medical, 2, 33; and narrative, 18–19, 110, 171–72, 179–80; schemata, 171; in stories, 10, 20–21, 214n7. *See also* discourse, and knowledge; storied knowledge
Korotana, Onkar, 214n9
Kurz, Demie, 139

labeling, 21–23, 65, 114, 139, 176
Labov, William, 13, 39–41, 144, 152, 153, 213n2, 213n4, 216n3; and diamond diagram,

5, 150; and observer's paradox, 43; and reportability, 21, 118, 144–45, 148, 160, 175, 179; on time, 72, 131, 162
LaFrance, Marianne, 158
Laing, Ronald D., 6, 45, 114
Lakoff, George, 69–70, 82, 88, 169, 217n1
Lakoff, Robin, 46, 217n1
Lamb, Sharon, 8, 140, 160
Langellier, Kristin M., 18
language: and culture, 11; as symbolic system, 16
Lanser, Susan S., 13
Larsen-Freeman, Diane, 151
Laurier, Eric, 72
Lawless, Elaine, 24, 99, 184
Lee, A. Russell, 6, 45, 114
Leech, Geoffrey N., 124
legislation, 37
levels of narrative analysis. *See* narrative context level; narrative discourse level
Levinson, Stephen C., 5, 46, 161
Lévi-Strauss, Claude, 94
life experiences, 133, 167. *See also* doctor-patient divide
life history research, 7, 58
Lind, E. Allan, 214n6
Linde, Charlotte, 26, 175, 214n8
listener, 5, 44, 103, 183. *See also* storyteller
literary studies and medicine, 182–83, 184, 217n2
Lloyd, Siobhan, 27
locatives, 82
logico-scientific mode. *See also* paradigmatic mode
Loseke, Donileen R., 22, 123, 140
Lyman, Stanford M., 103

macrolevel structures, 4, 8, 39, 93. *See also* microlevel structures
Marková, Ivana, 44
Mason, Jennifer, 37
Mattingly, Cheryl, 49
Maynard, Douglas W., 11, 22
Maynor, Natalie, 216n7
Mazza, Danielle, 30, 31
McCabe, Allyssa, 3, 5, 12
McEntyre, Marilyn Chandler, 217n2
McGarty, Craig, 9, 158
McKie, Linda, 37, 99

McLellan, M. Faith, 185
meaning, 3, 4
media and domestic violence, 37, 140, 152, 179
medical discourse, 17, 21, 62, 107, 116–17, 170, 182
medical ethics, 127
medical humanities, 183
medicine: history of, 33. *See also* narrative, and medicine
memory, 4, 20–21, 135, 153, 216n1. *See also* institutional memory
metaphor, 7, 68–73, 88–93, 176; cognitive account of, 69–70; and culture, 70; and medicine, 216–17n4; and narrative, 70–71; and spatiotemporal language, 71–73
Meyers, Marian, 140, 180
Mezey, Gill, 214n9
microlevel structures, 4, 6, 8, 39, 93, 114. *See also* macrolevel structures
Mildorf, Jarmila, 99
minimal narrative, 40. *See also* narrative
minimization, 138
miscommunication, 111, 213n2. *See also* communication problems
Mishler, Elliot G., 25
modalities, 80, 113, 123–24, 132, 137, 142–43, 149, 155, 162
Mooney, Jayne, 214n9
moral implications, 32–33, 50
motion verbs, 82
Müller, Frank, 162
Murch, Mervyn, 27, 215n3
myth, 94, 177; and domestic violence, 6, 8, 35–36, 106, 132, 154, 160, 167, 170, 175, 179, 216n6; of inadequacy, 116, 117–21, 176; of time, 99–103
mythologizing, 7, 102–3

narratee, 5, 42
narrative, 16, 18; as cognitive device, 12; as discursive device, 4, 12; and medicine, 6, 21–27, 98, 99, 181, 182, 183; practices, 7; production, 5, 15, 66; research, 13, 49, 173–74; syntax, 145–46. *See also* knowledge, in stories; minimal narrative; trajectories in narrative
narrative analysis, 2, 13, 19, 39–41, 54, 185
narrative clause typology, 40
narrative context level, 41, 43, 132

narrative discourse level, 41, 43
narrative frame, 5, 41, 42–44, 154
narrative framework. *See* narrative paradigm
narrative knowledge. *See* storied knowledge
narrative mode, 18–19, 214n7. *See also* paradigmatic mode; storied knowledge
narrativeness, 13
narrative paradigm, 3, 4, 7, 14–15, 173–74. *See also* scientific paradigm
narratology, 13, 213–14n5
narrator, 5, 103
narratory principle, 16
National Family Violence Survey, 29–30
National Health Service, x, 215–16n5
negators, 76, 115, 143
Nelson, Katherine, 146
noncompliance, 134
nondetection, 6, 31, 87, 95
nonresponse, 37
Norrick, Neal, xv, 5, 38, 144, 216n1
Nünning, Ansgar, 214n5
Nünning, Vera, 214n5

O'Barr, William M., 214n6
observer's paradox, 43
O'Connor, Blair, 33
ordering function of narrative, 4, 16, 110
orientation, 12, 40
Ortony, Andrew, 68

Pahl, Jan, 27
paradigmatic mode, 18, 214n7. *See also* narrative mode
Partnership Strategy, 37
passive construction, 83, 114, 127, 128–29, 151. *See also* active construction
path schema, 78–81, 88, 113, 169, 178
patiens, 127–28, 129, 135. See also *agens*
patient role. *See* sick role
patients' stories, 6, 17, 59, 62, 155, 183. *See also* doctors' stories; narrative, and medicine
pauses, 162, 163
Perception, 2, 5, 84, 158, 171, 214n7
performativity, 18, 173
Perkins, Jane, 25
perpetrator: images of, 109, 129, 151, 152, 180
Peterson, Eric E., 18
phatic features. *See* back channels; discourse markers; involvement

Phillipson, Herbert, 6, 45, 114
Pinker, Steven, 14
Pizzey, Erin, 28
point of view, 7, 109–10
politeness, 5, 46, 214n6
Polkinghorne, Donald, 4, 18–19, 121
Potter, Jonathan, 19
power and domestic violence, 8, 108
powerlessness, 32, 116, 117–21, 133–34, 176. *See also* inadequacy; myth, of inadequacy
practice environment, 38
presentation, 50; covert, 50, 51–52, 56; overt, 50, 51–52; standard, 54–58, 159. *See also* frequency
Prickett, Stephen, 70
Prince, Gerald, 214n5
privacy, 32, 87
professionalism, 26, 69, 112, 114, 117, 126–27, 170. *See also* expert knowledge; group, professional
Propp, Vladimir, 13
psychiatry and domestic violence, 27
psychology: discursive, 19; narrative, 18, 20; social, 9
psychosocial problems, 24, 127, 184
Ptacek, James, 103–4, 111, 176
purposive sampling, 37

qualitative research methods, 49, 174
Quirk, Randolph, 123, 162

Rachman, Stephen, 182–83
Radford, Andrew, 127
Radford, Jill, 214n9
reading the patient as text, 23, 182
record: medical, 95, 117, 126, 180, 182
repairs, 46, 65, 131. *See also* self-correction
repeat visits, 101
reportability, 40, 66, 118, 144–45, 171, 175, 179. *See also* evaluation
reportable events, 21, 150, 144–45, 151, 160, 169
research methodology, 36–38
resolution, 40
resource manual, 30–31
respondents, 37–38
responsibility, 34, 50, 81, 86, 112, 113–14, 143, 175. *See also* agency; roles
rewording, 23–24, 61–62, 182

rewriting. *See* rewording
Richardson, Jo, 27, 214n9
Riessman, Catherine Kohler, 49
Rigney, Ann, 18
ritual, 17
Robinson, John A., 12, 39
Rogers, L. Edna, 98–99
roles: social and professional, 41, 44, 45, 114, 126–27, 140, 176. *See also* professionalism
Rosewater, Lynne Bravo, 177
Rubin, Herbert, 44–45
Rubin, Irene, 44–45
rules for interaction, 5, 15
Ryan, Vicky, 30, 31

Sacks, Harvey, 44, 46, 216n1
Sack's Assignment Theorem, 144
sample narratives, 5, 6, 39, 57, 153. *See also* corpus
Sanders, Robert E., 19–20
Sapir, Edward, 11, 70
Sapir-Whorf hypothesis, 11, 213n1
Sarbin, Theodore R., 4, 16, 17
Schank, Roger C., 4, 18, 20–21, 39, 67, 153, 154
Schegloff, Emmanuel A., 5, 44, 46
Schiffrin, Deborah, 5, 17, 41, 119, 132, 135
Schornstein, Sherri L., 35, 75, 133, 161, 215n4, 217n2
Schütze, Fritz, 58–59
scientific paradigm, 14, 24, 33, 78, 117. *See also* narrative paradigm
Scott, Marvin B., 103
Scottish Executive, x, 37, 216n5
Scottish Needs Assessment Programme, 30
scripts, 20, 157, 171
second storying, 216n1
self-correction, 46, 155. *See also* repairs
self-criticism, 47, 121
self-monitoring, 43, 47, 131, 161
self-presentation, 98
sensitivity to domestic violence, 6, 78, 172
sequential organization of speech, 11, 40, 42
service provision, 27, 35
setting, 7, 72, 113. *See also* backgrounds; consultation room
severity, 78, 160
Shuy, Roger W., 25, 213n2
sick role, 34, 126–27, 139, 143

signs of abuse, 49–54, 66–67, 75, 78, 117, 157, 171–72. *See also* symptoms
silence, 6, 31, 161–63
Silverman, David, 25
situation. *See* context; interview, situation; storytelling situation
Smith, Philip, 6, 45
social class, 132, 133, 170, 216n6. *See also* sociodemographic factors
social control, 34
social problems, 3, 10–14, 112–13, 174
social sciences, 11
sociodemographic factors, 30, 46, 66. *See also* backgrounds; social class
sociolinguistic narrative analysis, 3, 26, 39, 184
sociolinguistics, 11, 13, 25
sociology of health and illness, 25
socionarratology, 3, 13–14, 120, 131
Solan, Lawrence M., 213n2
Sontag, Susan, 216–17n4
spacetime region, 71–72, 73, 178
spatiotemporal language, 7, 71–73, 79–80, 82, 85–86, 176, 178. *See also* metaphor, and spatiotemporal language; path schema
Spears, Russell, 9, 158
speech styles, 45, 132, 214n6
Spence, Donald P., 94, 177
spontaneous narratives, 39, 146, 157. *See also* interviewer-initiated narratives
Squier, Harriet A., 182–83, 184, 185
Stanko, Elizabeth A., 27
Stark, Evan, 139
status, 6, 84, 112
Stea, David, 71
Steinmetz, Suzanne K., 28, 29–30
stereotype formation, 9, 158
stereotypes, 9, 12, 111, 157–59, 170, 175. *See also* cliché
Stern, Josef, 68, 69
stigmatization, 6, 34, 84, 106, 138, 176. *See also* deviance
storied knowledge, 2, 4, 18–19, 21, 26, 32, 39, 93, 121, 152, 154, 157, 171, 178–79. *See also* knowledge
stories, 38–39; unfinished, 2, 6, 61–62, 75. *See also* doctors' stories; patients' stories; women's life stories
storing and indexing, 4, 20–21, 135, 153, 171

story logic, 10–11
storyteller, 5, 42–44. *See also* listener
storytelling, 14, 17, 103, 144–145. *See also* narrative
storytelling situation, 97–98, 157
Straus, Murray A., 28, 29–30
Strauss, Anselm, 58
Streit Olness, Gloria, 15
Strong, Philip, 17, 87–89, 125, 178
structure: social, 11, 12, 213n3
Sugg, Nancy Kathleen, 32, 95
suspense, 149, 152, 162
symptoms, 49–54, 56, 78, 117. *See also* signs of abuse
syntactic parallelism, 48, 74, 135, 152, 168
Szokolszky, Agnes, 68

taboos, 6, 161, 163, 178
talk-in-interaction, 5, 6, 19, 47–48
Tannen, Deborah, 25, 41, 48, 108, 156, 175
Tayside Women and Violence Group, 27, 215n11
teaching module, 182–83, 184–85
te Molder, Hedwig, 19
temporal juncture, 40
tense, 66, 131, 134, 148, 162, 170
thematic roles, 127–28, 129
theta theory, 124, 127
Tiersma, Peter, 213n2
time, 32, 37, 77, 95–103; in narrative, 72, 131, 162. *See also* myth, of time; tense
Titscher, Stefan, 16
Todd, Alexandra Dundas, 25
Tolliver, Joyce, 13
Toolan, Michael, 13
training, 8, 111, 181
trajectories in narrative, 6, 7, 57, 58–67
transactions, 19, 110, 126
transcription of data, 38, 216n7
Trinch, Shonna, 23–24, 26, 61–62, 129, 163, 175, 214–15n10
Turner, Terence, 68–69
turn taking, 44, 46, 144–45
type and token analysis, 50–51

Ulatowska, Hanna K., 15

van Dijk, Teun, 3
variables, 46

vectors: spatial, 82, 86, 178, 216n3
victimization, 22–23, 30, 130, 137, 140, 143, 159, 176
victims, 8; images of, 22, 74, 137, 140, 148, 160, 178, 180
violence against women, 28, 30

Wales, Katie, 161
Waletzky, Joshua, 13, 39–41, 144, 152, 153, 213n4
Walker, Val, 27, 215n3
Wallat, Cynthia, 25
Warshaw, Carole, 27, 95
Wellberry, D. E., 68
wellness-illness divide. *See* doctor-patient divide
West, Candace, 25
Whalen, Jack, 12, 217n1
Whalen, Marylin R., 12, 217n1
Whorf, Benjamin Lee, 11, 70
Widdicombe, Sue, 17

Williamson, Emma, 30, 31, 32, 34, 35, 36, 111, 138, 139, 140, 164, 172, 178, 184, 215n3, 215n4
Willson, Pam, 29
Wilson, Claudia, 214n9
Wilson, Thomas P., 11
witness, 143
Wodak, Ruth, 99
Wolfson, Nessa, 43
Women's Aid groups, 28
women's life stories, 61, 143, 180
World Bank, ix
World Health Organization, 215n4

Young, D., 215n4
Young, Katherine, 44, 57, 73, 117, 126, 178
Yzerbyt, Vincent Y., 9, 158

Zero Tolerance campaign, 179, 217n1
Zimmerman, Don H., 12, 213n3, 217n1

In the Frontiers of Narrative series:

Story Logic: Problems and Possibilities of Narrative
by David Herman

Handbook of Narrative Analysis
by Luc Herman and Bart Varvaeck

Spaces of the Mind: Narrative and Community in the American West
by Elaine A. Jahner

Talk Fiction: Literature and the Talk Explosion
by Irene Kacandes

Storying Domestic Violence
Constructions and Stereotypes of Abuse in the Discourse of General Practitioners
by Jarmila Mildorf

Fictional Minds
by Alan Palmer

Narrative across Media: The Languages of Storytelling
edited by Marie-Laure Ryan